THE ANMOL JEEVAN FOUNDATION ACCELERATED RECOVERY PROGRAM

THE ANMOL JEEVAN FOUNDATION ACCELERATED RECOVERY & RELAPSE MANAGEMENT PROGRAM

© 2024 – ANMOL JEEVAN FOUNDATION PERMANENT HOSPITAL REGISTRATION NO. 5 / 2023 – PROPRIETARY AWARENESS & TRAINING MATERIAL FOR RECOVERING DRUG / SEX / CYBER / PORN ADDICTS, ALCOHOLICS, GAMBLERS, PSYCHIATRIC ILLNESS AND PERSONALITY DISORDERS

 ANMOL JEEVAN FOUNDATION – PSYCHIATRIC HOSPITAL & NURSING HOME SPECIALIZED IN DE-ADDICTION THERAPY, MENTAL ILLNESS AND PSYCHIATRIC CARE – PERMANENT REGISTRATION NO. 5/2023

FOR THOSE FAMILIES … WHO HAVE AN ALCOHOLIC, ADDICT, GAMBLER, ANY PERSON SUFFERING FROM MENTAL OR PSYCHIATRIC ILLNESS, OR PERSONALITY DISORDERS IN THEIR LIVES
45 DAY – ACCELERATED RECOVERY PROGRAM

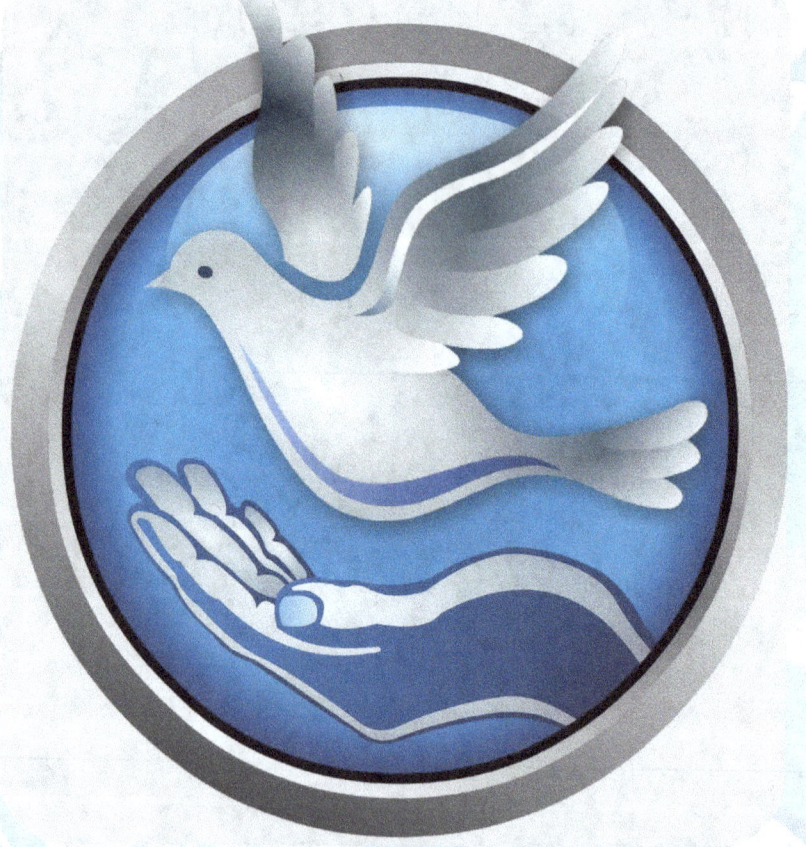

DO YOU HAVE SOMEONE (THAT YOU LOVE) IN YOUR LIFE WHO IS CONSUMING ALCOHOL OR DRUGS – THAT SEEMS TO BE OUT OF HIS CONTROL?

DID YOU KNOW THAT ANY OF <u>ALCOHOL OR DRUG ADDICTION IS A DISEASE</u>? – AND THAT THIS IS A LIFE-LONG CHRONIC CONDITION, WHICH LEADS TO LONG-TERM SOCIO-PSYCHO-ECONOMIC EFFECTS?

<u>THIS IS A SELF-HELP GUIDE FOR THOSE FAMILIES SEEKING TO HELP A "VERY SICK PERSON", AND OVERCOME ANY OF THESE MALADIES</u>

© 2023 - A WELLBEING GUIDE FOR THE FAMILIES & FRIENDS OF ALCOHOL, DRUG, SEX ADDICTS, AND COMPULSIVE GAMBLERS BY THE ANMOL JEEVAN FOUNDATION™
ANMOLJEEVANWELNESS@GMAIL.COM WWW.ANMOLWELNESS.ORG
+91 915807 1666 / 915807 9666 & +91 8080 8989 41/42

 ANMOL JEEVAN FOUNDATION – PSYCHIATRIC HOSPITAL & NURSING HOME SPECIALIZED IN DE-ADDICTION THERAPY, MENTAL ILLNESS AND PSYCHIATRIC CARE – PERMANENT REGISTRATION NO. 5/2023

SEEK HELP, BEFORE ITS TOO LATE – WE ARE HERE FOR YOU.

ALCOHOL, DRUGS, GAMBLING, SEX OR ANY OTHER SUBSTANCE AND NON-SUBSTANCE ABUSE, OR ANY MENTAL ILLNESS …

DO NOT STRUGGLE ALONE! – WE ARE WITH YOU!

REACH OUT TO US 24 X 7 X 365

ANMOL JEEVAN FOUNDATION PSYCHIATRIC HOSPITAL

RAJDOOT WADI, PURNUKPADA, VAJRESHWARI ROAD,

SHIRAVLI, POST PAROL, VIRAR (EAST),

TALUKA – VASAI, DISTRICT – PALGHAR – 401 303.

MAHARASHTRA, INDIA.

ANMOLJEEVANWELNESS@GMAIL.COM

WWW.ANMOLWELNESS.ORG

+91 915807 1666 / 915807 9666 &

+91 8080 8989 41/42

ALSO FIND AND CONNECT WITH US ON SOCIAL MEDIA – FACEBOOK AND INSTAGRAM

 ANMOL JEEVAN FOUNDATION – PSYCHIATRIC HOSPITAL & NURSING HOME SPECIALIZED IN DE-ADDICTION THERAPY, MENTAL ILLNESS AND PSYCHIATRIC CARE – PERMANENT REGISTRATION NO. 5/2023

WHAT IS THE ANMOL JEEVAN ACCELERATED RECOVERY PROGRAM?

ANMOL JEEVAN FOUNDATION OFFERS AN UNIQUE 45 DAY RECOVERY PLAN THAT IS BASED ON BEST PRACTICES OF THE DIAGNOSTIC AND STATISTICAL MANUAL OF MENTAL DISORDERS (DSM-IV), THE GORSKI-CENAPS© MODEL OF RECOVERY AND RELAPSE PREVENTION, CENTRE FOR SUBSTANCE ABUSE TREATMENT (CSAT, USA), THE HAZELDEN DEVELOPMENTAL MODEL OF RECOVERY (DMR), THE 12 STEPS OF ALCOHOLICS / NARCOTICS ANONYMOUS (AA / NA), AND THE EXPERIENCE OF THOUSANDS OF RECOVERING ADDICTS AROUND THE WORLD.

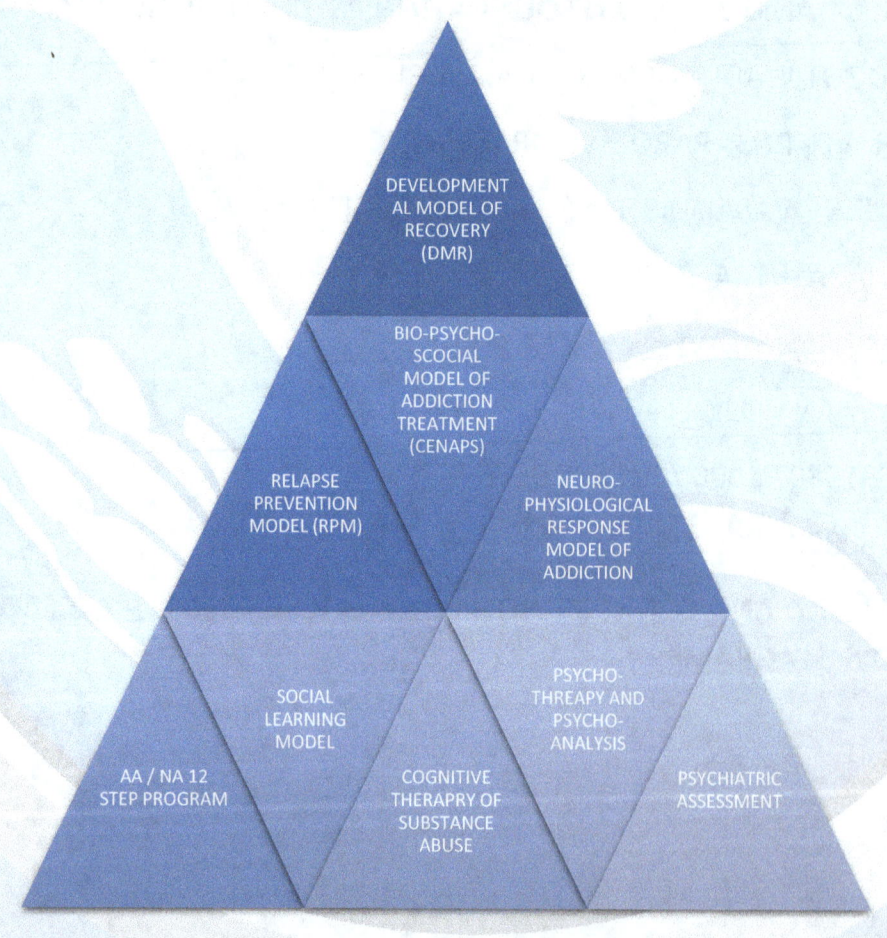

© 2023 - A WELLBEING GUIDE FOR THE FAMILIES & FRIENDS OF ALCOHOL, DRUG, SEX ADDICTS, AND COMPULSIVE GAMBLERS BY THE ANMOL JEEVAN FOUNDATION™
ANMOLJEEVANWELNESS@GMAIL.COM WWW.ANMOLWELNESS.ORG
+91 915807 1666 / 915807 9666 & +91 8080 8989 41/42

 ANMOL JEEVAN FOUNDATION – PSYCHIATRIC HOSPITAL & NURSING HOME SPECIALIZED IN DE-ADDICTION THERAPY, MENTAL ILLNESS AND PSYCHIATRIC CARE – PERMANENT REGISTRATION NO. 5/2023

WE ADOPT A **3 DIMENSIONAL APPROACH** TO TREATMENT OF THE ADDICT PATIENTS –

- PRE-TREATMENT DETOXIFICATION
- PHYSICAL & MENTAL ASSESSMENT
- CONTINUOUS COUNSELLING, PSYCHOLOGICAL ASSESSMENT & 12 STEP PROGRAM

THE 45 DAYS ARE STRATEGICALLY BROKEN DOWN INTO 4 PHASES –

WEEKS 1 & 2

- PATIENT BACKGROUND AND HISTORY
- FAMILY COUNSELLING - ADDICTION DISEASE CONCEPT, TREATMENT PATTERN AND CONCERNS
- PATIENT DETOXIFICATION
- PHYSIOLOGICAL MEDICAL ASSESSMENT
- ECG
- PATHOLOGICAL INVESTIGATIONS
- PSYCHIATRIC EVALUATION
- PHARMACOLOGICAL REGIME
- DIET DETERMINATION
- PHYSICAL WORKOUT AND GROUP THERAPY
- FAMILY FEEDBACK - BIO-PSYCHO-SOCIAL BY PSYCHIATRIST AND COUNSELLOR

WEEKS 3 & 4

- PSYCHIATRIC RE-EVALUATION
- INDIVIDUAL COUNSELLING AND THERAPY BASED ON PSYCHOLOGICAL ASSESSMENTS
- AA / NA STEP WORKING WITH DEDICATED COUNSELLOR
- ASSIGNMENTS BASED ON IQ AND APTITUDE
- PATIENT PROGRESS TRACKING & FAMILY FEEDBACK VIA VIDEO CONFERENCING

WEEK 4 & 5

- ALIGNMENT OF PATIENT TO THE 12 STEP PROGRAM
- PARTICIPATION IN THE IN-HOUSE AA/NA MEETINGS
- PERSONAL COUNSELLING BASED ON PSYCHOLOGICAL EVALUATION
- FAMILY VISIT & FACTUAL CONFRONTATION (FCC)
- ADVANCED STEP WORKING, AND SPIRITUAL DEVELOPMENT

WEEK 6 - DISCHARGE

- FCC OUTPUT BASED COUNSELLING
- REASSESSMENT OF PATIENT READINESS AND WILLINGNESS
- PREPARING FOR THE OUTSIDE WORLD - ACCEPT NEW REALITIES
- RELAPSE MANAGEMENT PROGRAM
- COUNSELLOR SIGN OFF
- JOINT COUNSELLING SESSION - FAMILY & PATIENT RE-INTEGRATION
- GUIDANCE ON MAINTENANCE PHASE - AA / NA + AL-ANON / NAR-ANON OR ALA-TEEN MEETINGS

© 2023 - A WELLBEING GUIDE FOR THE FAMILIES & FRIENDS OF ALCOHOL, DRUG, SEX ADDICTS, AND COMPULSIVE GAMBLERS BY THE ANMOL JEEVAN FOUNDATION™
ANMOLJEEVANWELNESS@GMAIL.COM WWW.ANMOLWELNESS.ORG
+91 915807 1666 / 915807 9666 & +91 8080 8989 41/42

 ANMOL JEEVAN FOUNDATION – PSYCHIATRIC HOSPITAL & NURSING HOME SPECIALIZED IN DE-ADDICTION THERAPY, MENTAL ILLNESS AND PSYCHIATRIC CARE – PERMANENT REGISTRATION NO. 5/2023

PHYSIOLOGICAL EVALUATIONS	PHYSIATRIC EVALUATION	PSYCHOLOGICAL EVALATIONS	PERSONAL COUNSELLING
• COVID TESTING • DRUG / ALCOHOL TESTING • MEDICAL ASSESSMENT • ECG • FULL BLOOD & URINE PANEL • LIVER, KIDNEY FUNCTION TESTS • THYROID TESTS • BLOOD COUNT ANALYSIS • SUGAR CONTROL ANALYSIS	• MENTAL AND EMOTIONAL STATE • PAIN MANAGMENT • (SUBSTANCE) CRAVING CONTROL • MOOD ANALYSIS • PHARMA SUBSTITUTION / REPLACEMENT	• MMPI/ MCMI • HTP • TAT • RORSHARC / INK BLOT • K10 - DASS 21 - DEPRESSION / ANXIETY ANALYSIS • DAST • AUDIT • PERSONALITY ANALYSIS • AWARE RELAPSE ANALSYS	• PATIENT ALIGNMENT STATUS & GENERAL WELL-BEING • PATIENT AUTOBIOGRAPHY - LIFE HIGHLIGHT ANALYSIS • ANGER - FEAR - GUILT ANALYSIS • AA / NA 12 STEP WORKING • DAILY THOUGHT- EMOTION & CHARACTER DEFECT INVENTORY

THE **POST-DISCHARGE FOLLOW UP** COMPROMISES OF –

- 1 CLIENT VISIT + 48 HOUR STAY AT THE CENTRE – TO REVISIT THE 12 STEP RECOVERY PROGRAM WITH THE COUNSELLOR, AS WELL AS A REVISION OF THE RELAPSE PREVENTION PROGRAM (RPP). THIS IS DONE 15 DAYS POST DISCHARGE.
- 2 CLIENT + FAMILY VISITS TO THE CENTRE – FOR A PSYCHIATRIC FOLLOW UP, AND TO SEEK ADVISE FROM THE COUNSELLORS ON MAINTAINING RECOVERY. THESE VISITS ARE TO BE SCHEDULED BETWEEN 30-60 DAYS POST DISCHARGE, BY TAKING A PRIOR APPOINTMENT FROM THE ADMINISTRATION DEPARTMENT.

© 2023 - A WELLBEING GUIDE FOR THE FAMILIES & FRIENDS OF ALCOHOL, DRUG, SEX ADDICTS, AND COMPULSIVE GAMBLERS BY THE ANMOL JEEVAN FOUNDATION™
ANMOLJEEVANWELNESS@GMAIL.COM WWW.ANMOLWELNESS.ORG
+91 915807 1666 / 915807 9666 & +91 8080 8989 41/42

ANMOL JEEVAN FOUNDATION – PSYCHIATRIC HOSPITAL & NURSING HOME SPECIALIZED IN DE-ADDICTION THERAPY, MENTAL ILLNESS AND PSYCHIATRIC CARE – PERMANENT REGISTRATION NO. 5/2023

WHAT DOES ANMOL JEEVAN PROMISE TO OFFER?

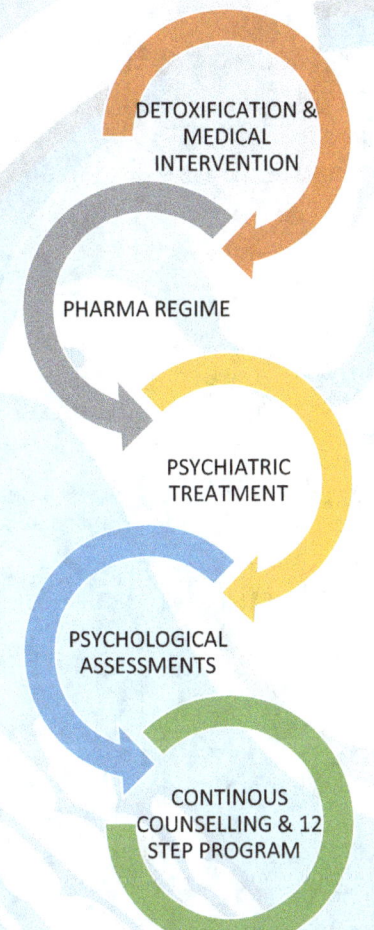

AT ANMOL JEEVAN WE FIRMLY BELIEVE THAT –

- NO TWO ADDICTS ARE THE SAME, THERE IS NO ONE-SIZE-FITS-ALL TREATMENT
- EVERY ADDICT COMES TO US WITH A UNIQUE PAST, MENTAL RESERVATIONS AND EMOTIONAL STATE OF MIND
- EVERY ADDICT DESERVES RESPECT AND A HELPING HAND – HE IS NOT TO BE DRAGGED THROUGH THE MUD, OR SHAMED FOR THIS PAST
- HOPE-FILLED ADDICTS AND STRONG FAMILIES ARE MOST LIKELY TO INTEGRATE AND PROSPER
- THE REHAB SHOULD BE JUST LIKE A "HOME, AWAY FROM HOME"

WE START OUR ADMISSION PROCEDURE WITH THE PROCESS OF "**DETOXIFICATION**" AND THOROUGH **PHYSIOLOGICAL AND PATHOLOGICAL INVESTIGATIONS** – THUS DETERMINING THE FITNESS OF THE PATIENT TO START THE PROGRAM. WE ALLOW AS MUCH TIME AS THE PATIENT NEEDS TO STAND HIS GROUND FIRMLY, AND BE ACCUSTOMED TO THE NEW CONDITIONS OF THE REHAB.

THE PHARMACOLOGICAL (MEDICINES) REGIME IS FINALIZED AFTER A DETAILED PSYCHIATRIC ASSESSMENT. WE ASCERTAIN MENTAL AILMENTS AND DISORDERS, OR ANY OTHER "SPECIAL NEEDS" OF THE PATIENT. **THE DIET AND PHYSICAL ACTIVITY PLAN OF THE PATIENT IS ALSO FINALIZED BY THE MEDICAL TEAMS.**

WE OFFER WHOLESOME MEALS THAT ARE DESIGNED TO FULFIL THE NUTRITION AND NOURISHMENT NEEDS EVERY PATIENT. "SPECIAL NEEDS" PATIENTS, DIABETICS OR THOSE SUFFERING FROM LIVER AND DIGESTIVE AILMENTS ARE PROVIDED WITH MEALS TO SUIT THEIR NEEDS AND INTAKE IS MONITORED BY THE ONSITE MEDICAL TEAM. SUMMARY OF OUR MEAL PROGRAM WOULD BE –

© 2023 - A WELLBEING GUIDE FOR THE FAMILIES & FRIENDS OF ALCOHOL, DRUG, SEX ADDICTS, AND COMPULSIVE GAMBLERS BY THE ANMOL JEEVAN FOUNDATION™
ANMOLJEEVANWELNESS@GMAIL.COM WWW.ANMOLWELNESS.ORG
+91 915807 1666 / 915807 9666 & +91 8080 8989 41/42

 **ANMOL JEEVAN FOUNDATION – PSYCHIATRIC HOSPITAL & NURSING HOME SPECIALIZED IN DE-ADDICTION THERAPY, MENTAL ILLNESS AND PSYCHIATRIC CARE – PERMANENT REGISTRATION NO. 5/2023**

- VARIETY OF VEGETARIAN & NON-VEGETARIAN MEALS
- EGGS – BOILED OR FRIED TWICE A WEEK
- SPECIALITY FOOD – CHINESE, CONTINENTAL AND INDIAN OCCASIONALLY
- JAIN MEALS
- MILK (WITH BOURNVITA / HORLICKS) – TWICE A DAY
- DIGESTIVE BISCUITS / PACKAGED SNACKS FOR IN-ROOM CONSUMPTION
- DAILY EVENING REFRESHMENTS WITH TEA OR COFFEE
- SEASONAL FRUITS / FRUIT JUICES / SOFT DRINKS
- CAKES AND DESERTS ON SPECIAL OCCASIONS AND FESTIVALS

ALL MEALS ARE FRESHLY COOKED AND SERVED.

RECREATION AND GROOMING ACTIVITIES INCLUDE –

- OUTDOOR SPORTS SUCH AS VOLLEYBALL, CRICKET, BADMINTON
- INDOOR SPORTS SUCH AS CAROM, CHESS, BILLIARDS / POOL
- HAIR SALON AND SPA – HAIR CUTTING / DYING / STYLING, SHAVING, AND MASSAGE
- LIBRARY – RICH IN AA / NA LITERATURE, FICTION AND NON-FICTION BOOKS, SELF HELP GUIDES, NOVELS, INSPIRATIONAL AND MOTIVATIONAL TEXTS
- MUSICAL INSTRUMENTS
- PERIODIC FUN ACTIVITIES LIKE HOUSIE, MUSICAL CHAIRS, DANCE
- YOGA, PT EXERCISES, STRETCHING, CHAIR / SITTING EXERCISES, MEDITATION AND ZUMBA – EITHER IS DONE ON A DAILY BASIS

THE ROOM AND INFRASTRUCTURE FACILITIES INCLUDE –

- SPACIOUS AND AIR-CONDITIONED ROOMS
- ATTACHED WASHROOM PER ROOM EQUIPPED WITH GEYSER AND SHOWER
- DAILY LAUNDRY PICK UP / DROP SERVICE
- BASIC TOILETRIES ARE PROVIDED IN-CENTRE
- DAILY ROOM SANITATION AND MOSQUITO FOGGING
- HOT-COLD DRINKING WATER DISPENSER
- TV WITH TATA SKY DTH
- READING AND STUDY TABLE
- 24X7 CCTV SURVEILLANCE, SECURITY TEAMS WITH WALKY-TALKIES
- ONE STAFF MEMBER PER ROOM
- RESIDENT MEDICAL OFFICER AND PHARMACIST

WE HAVE A TEAM OF EXPERT PROFESSIONALS TO ENSURE OVERALL RECOVERY AND MONITOR THE PROGRESS OF EVERY PATIENT –

- THE DETOXIFICATION CENTRE IS EQUIPPED WITH ECG MACHINES AND RESPIRATORY EQUIPMENT

© 2023 - A WELLBEING GUIDE FOR THE FAMILIES & FRIENDS OF ALCOHOL, DRUG, SEX ADDICTS, AND COMPULSIVE GAMBLERS BY THE ANMOL JEEVAN FOUNDATION™
ANMOLJEEVANWELNESS@GMAIL.COM WWW.ANMOLWELNESS.ORG
+91 915807 1666 / 915807 9666 & +91 8080 8989 41/42

 ANMOL JEEVAN FOUNDATION – PSYCHIATRIC HOSPITAL & NURSING HOME SPECIALIZED IN DE-ADDICTION THERAPY, MENTAL ILLNESS AND PSYCHIATRIC CARE – PERMANENT REGISTRATION NO. 5/2023

- IN-CENTRE PHARMACY FOR ADMINISTERING MEDICINES, INJECTABLE DRUGS AND 24X7 EMERGENCY RESPONSE IN CASE OF PATIENT DISTRESS
- DEDICATED AMBULANCE FOR EMERGENCY PATIENT TRANSPORT – AVAILABLE 24X7 ON PREMISE
- BEST IN CLASS PSYCHIATRIC DOCTORS ATTACHED
- TEAM OF PSYCHOLOGISTS TO A WIDE PANEL OF PSYCHOLOGICAL ASSESSMENTS
- DEDICATED COUNSELLORS ASSIGNED TO EACH PATIENT, WHO GUIDE THEM THROUGH THE 12 STEP PROGRAM AND ASSIST THEM IN EVERY STEP OF DE-ADDICT AND RELAPSE PREVENTION

STRATEGIC ALLIANCES WITH HOSPITALS, PATHOLOGY LABORATORIES AND MENTAL TREATMENT FACILITIES FOR –

- X-RAYS
- BLOOD / URINE / COVID TESTS
- ECT – ELECTRO OR CHEMICAL IMBALANCE TREATMENTS
- DENTAL TREATMENT
- OPHTHALMOLOGIST (EYE DOCTOR) AND DERMATOLOGIST (SKIN DOCTOR)
- BONE-MUSCLE TREATMENTS, FRACTURE PLASTERING ETC ...

THE DAILY ROUTINE OF PATIENTS STRICTLY MONITORED BY THE IN-HOUSE STAFF. STARTING FROM BASIC HYGIENE CHECKS TO TRACKING PROGRESS IN THE 12 STEP PROGRAM IS THOROUGHLY TRACKED.

THE ADMINISTRATION STAFF KEEPS THE FAMILY UPDATED ON THE PROGRESS OF THE PATIENT, AND WHEN SOME MILESTONES ARE CROSSED. THE DOCTOR AND PSYCHIATRIST ALSO ROUTINELY UPDATE THE FAMILY ON THE PATIENTS WELL-BEING.

THE DEDICATED COUNSELLOR WORKS ALONGSIDE THE FAMILY MEMBERS TO CONDUCT FAMILY MEETINGS AND CONFRONTATIONS, BASED ON THE RECOVERY PROGRESS OF THE PATIENT.

THE FAMILY IS FREE TO CALL THE CENTRE TO SEEK UPDATES OR PROVIDE ANY ADDITIONAL CASE INFORMATION, BASED ON A CONVENIENT TIME SLOT FIXED WITH THE ADMINISTRATION OFFICE.

ANMOLJEEVANWELNESS@GMAIL.COM

WWW.ANMOLWELNESS.ORG

+91 915807 1666 / 915807 9666 &

+91 8080 8989 41/42

© 2023 - A WELLBEING GUIDE FOR THE FAMILIES & FRIENDS OF ALCOHOL, DRUG, SEX ADDICTS, AND COMPULSIVE GAMBLERS BY THE ANMOL JEEVAN FOUNDATION™
ANMOLJEEVANWELNESS@GMAIL.COM WWW.ANMOLWELNESS.ORG
+91 915807 1666 / 915807 9666 & +91 8080 8989 41/42

ANMOL JEEVAN FOUNDATION – PSYCHIATRIC HOSPITAL & NURSING HOME SPECIALIZED IN DE-ADDICTION THERAPY, MENTAL ILLNESS AND PSYCHIATRIC CARE – PERMANENT REGISTRATION NO. 5/2023

FEES, CHARGES, TERMS & CONDITIONS –

THE 45 DAY ACCELERATED RECOVERY PROGRAM IS AN ALL-INCLUSIVE PACKAGE, WITH SOME ITEMS THAT ARE SEPARATELY PAYABLE –

45 DAY PACKAGE ENROLMENT REQUIRES AN ADVANCE PAYMENT OF INR 60,000/-. THIS FEE IS PAYABLE FULLY IN ADVANCE. THESE FEES ARE NON-REFUNDABLE ON A PRORATED BASIS, AND THE ENTIRE PROGRAM MAY BE RE-ENROLLED BY PAYING THE SAME AMOUNT.

THIS FEE INCLUDES –

- THE DETOXIFICATION FEE + ONE ECG
- RESIDENT DOCTOR CHARGES
- PSYCHIATRIC DOCTOR CHARGES
- ONE ROUND OF BLOOD PANEL TESTING – (COMPLETE BLOOD COUNT, LIVER FUNCTION TEST, KIDNEY FUNCTION TEST, BLOOD-SUGAR TESTING & THYROID FUNCTION TEST)
- NARCO-URINE PLATE ANALYSIS
- ACCOMMODATION (AS DESCRIBED ABOVE)
- 3 SQUARE MEALS, AND EVENING SNACKS. SPECIAL MEALS ON WEEKENDS AND HOLIDAYS
- IN-ROOM SNACKS FOR ODD HOUR HUNGER PANGS
- LAUNDRY SERVICE
- ACCESS TO ALL AMENITIES SUCH AS THE SALON & SPA, GYMNASIUM, LIBRARY AND SPORTS / GAMES FACILITIES
- STATIONARY, STEP WORKING BOOK CHARGES, LAEFLETS, BOOKS AND INFORMATIONAL MATERIAL
- PSYCHOTHERAPY SESSIONS
- PSYCHOLOGICAL TESTING, REPORTING AND ANALYSIS
- COUNSELLOR & GUEST LECTURES
- INDIVIDUAL & GROUP COUNSELLING / THERAPY SESSIONS
- BASIC TOILETRIES (COMPRISING OF SHOWER GEL, SHAMPOO, TOOTHBRUSH / PASTE, DEODORANT)

ADDITIONAL CHARGES SHALL BE LEVIED FOR –

- ALL PRESCRIBED PHARMACEUTICALS, MEDICINES, CREAMS, LOTIONS ETC.
- PATIENT PICKUP MAY BE ARRANGED BY ANMOL JEEVAN, BUT SHALL BE CHARGED SEPARATELY
- ANY ADDITIONAL TESTS REQUIRED APART FROM THE ONES MENTIONED ABOVE
- X-RAYS, MRI, OR OTHER BLOOD, URINE AND STOOL TESTS
- ANY NON-PSYCHIATRIC CONSULTATION SUCH AS (BUT NOT LIMITED TO) ORTHOPAEDIC, OPHTHALMOLOGIST, DENTIST, UROLOGIST OR HEPATOLOGIST. ANMOL JEEVAN HAS STRATEGIC TIE-UPS FOR SUCH TESTS OR SPECIALIST CONSULTATIONS – THEY SHALL BE CHARGED ON ACTUALS
- ADDITIONAL CHARGES ON ACTUALS FOR SPECIFIC DEMANDS FOR TOILETRIES BEYOND THOSE MENTIONED ABOVE
- SPECIALITY FOOD TO BE ORDERED FROM OUTSIDE SHALL BE CHARGED ON ACTUALS
- AMBULANCE FEES FOR TRANSPORTATION SHALL BE SEPARATELY CHARGED

© 2023 - A WELLBEING GUIDE FOR THE FAMILIES & FRIENDS OF ALCOHOL, DRUG, SEX ADDICTS, AND COMPULSIVE GAMBLERS BY THE ANMOL JEEVAN FOUNDATION™
ANMOLJEEVANWELNESS@GMAIL.COM WWW.ANMOLWELNESS.ORG
+91 915807 1666 / 915807 9666 & +91 8080 8989 41/42

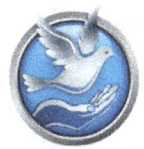 © 2024 – ANMOL JEEVAN FOUNDATION – PROPRIETARY AWARENESS & TRAINING MATERIAL FOR RECOVERING DRUG / SEX / CYBER / PORN ADDICTS, ALCOHOLICS, GAMBLERS, PSYCHIATRIC ILLNESS AND PERSONALITY DISORDERS.

TABLE OF CONTENTS –

TABLE OF CONTENTS – 2
AM I AN ADDICT? 3
THE ALCOHOLICS ANONYMOUS 20 ITEM QUESTIONNAIRE 5
HARMFUL EFFECTS AND CONSEQUENCES OF ADDICTION IN MY LIFE 7
WHAT IS THE NATURE OF MY MENTAL OBSESSION, PHYSICAL COMPULSION AND SPIRITUAL BANKRUPTCY? 16
AUTOBIOGRAPHY 22
STEP ONE 23
STEP ONE TEST 52
STEP TWO 54
STEP TWO TEST 80
STEP THREE 81
STEP THREE TEST 97
FINANCIAL MISMANAGEMENT INVENTORY 99

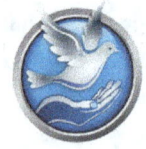

© 2024 – ANMOL JEEVAN FOUNDATION – PROPRIETARY AWARENESS & TRAINING MATERIAL FOR RECOVERING DRUG / SEX / CYBER / PORN ADDICTS, ALCOHOLICS, GAMBLERS, PSYCHIATRIC ILLNESS AND PERSONALITY DISORDERS.

AM I AN ADDICT?

#	QUESTION	YES	NO
1	DOES ADDICTION OR GAMBLING CAUSE YOU TO LOSE TIME FROM HIS ACTUAL JOB?		
2	IS THIS COMPULSIVE ADDICTION, GAMBLING OR SPENDING CAUSING FAMILY DISTURBANCES?		
3	DO YOUR SPENDING HABITS OR BETTING AFFECTING YOUR SOCIAL STATURE / REPUTATION?		
4	IS THE ADDICTION OR GAMBLING CAUSING YOU, OR YOUR FAMILY FINANCIAL DIFFICULTIES?		
5	DOES YOU FEEL GUILTY AFTER CONSUMING ALCOHOL AND DRUGS OR ENGAGING IN GAMBLING?		
6	DOES YOU IMMEDIATELY FEEL A STRONG URGE TO DRINK OR USE DRUGS, WHEN THE EFFECT WEARS OFF?		
7	DOES YOU CONTINUE TO DRINK, DO DRUGS OR GAMBLE UNTIL HIS OR YOUR VERY LAST RUPEE?		
8	HAVE YOU HAD TO SELL ANYTHING TO MEET YOUR DRINKING, DRUG OR GAMBLING URGE?		
9	HAVE YOU COMMITTED ANY ILLEGAL ACTS OR HURT OTHERS TO FEED YOUR ADDICTION OR GAMBLING HABITS?		
10	HAVE YOU CONSIDERED SELF-HARM OR EXPERIENCED EXTREME LOSS OF HOPE DUE TO YOUR HABITS OF DRINKING, DRUGS OR GAMBLING?		

KINDLY ANSWER THE ABOVE CHECKLIST WITH COMPLETE HONESTY. YOU SHALL MOST LIKELY BE ENLIGHTNED WITH THE FINDINGS. HERE IS A 10-POINT ADDICTION QUESTIONNAIRE

REMEMBER – A "MAYBE" ALSO MEANS A "YES"!

PLEASE BEAR MIND THAT THE ADDICT HIMSELF, AND HIS FAMILY SHALL BEGIN TO OVERCOME THEIR PROBLEMS, IF AND ONLY YOU COMPLETELY HONEST WITH

THE ANMOL JEEVAN ACCELERATED RECOVERY & RELAPSE MANAGEMENT PROGRAM™

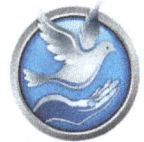 © 2024 – ANMOL JEEVAN FOUNDATION – PROPRIETARY AWARENESS & TRAINING MATERIAL FOR RECOVERING DRUG / SEX / CYBER / PORN ADDICTS, ALCOHOLICS, GAMBLERS, PSYCHIATRIC ILLNESS AND PERSONALITY DISORDERS.

YOURSELF, FIRST. AND, <u>THAT YOU ARE WILLING TO "ACCEPT" THE PROBLEM AND SEEK HELP ACCORDINGLY.</u>

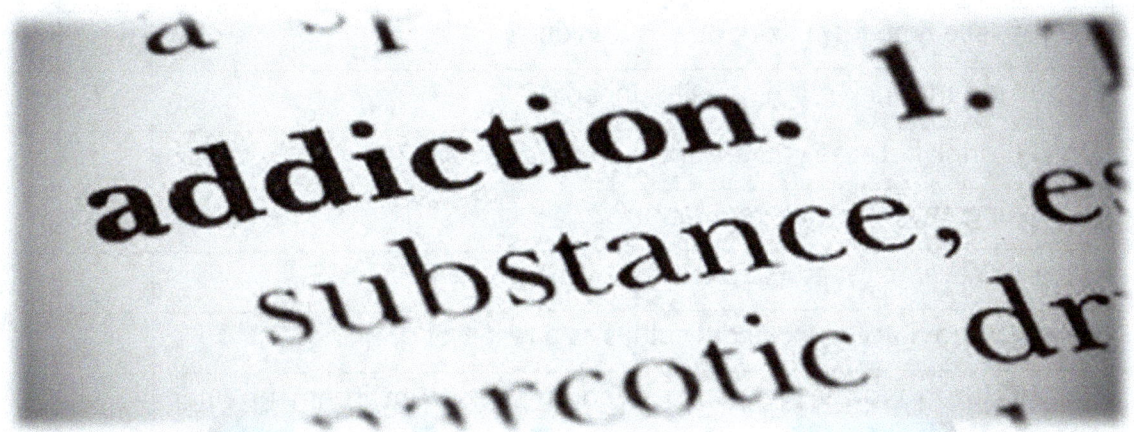

RESULTS –

- IF YOU'VE ANSWERED AT LEAST 2 AS "YES" – <u>THEN YOU MAY OR MAY NOT BE AN ADDICT</u>
- IF YOU'VE ANSWERED AT LEAST 4 AS "YES" – <u>THEN THERE ARE VERY HIGH CHANCES THAT YOU ARE AN ADDICT</u>
- IF YOU'VE ANSWERED MORE THAN 4 AS "YES" – <u>THEN YOU ARE CERTAINLY AN ADDICT; AND SHOULD BE SEEKING HELP IMMEDIATELY</u>

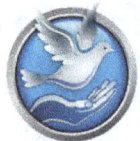

© 2024 – ANMOL JEEVAN FOUNDATION – PROPRIETARY AWARENESS & TRAINING MATERIAL FOR RECOVERING DRUG / SEX / CYBER / PORN ADDICTS, ALCOHOLICS, GAMBLERS, PSYCHIATRIC ILLNESS AND PERSONALITY DISORDERS.

THE ALCOHOLICS ANONYMOUS 20 ITEM QUESTIONNAIRE

Sr.	Question	Yes	No
1	Do you lose time from work due to drinking?		
2	Is drinking making your home life unhappy?		
3	Do you drink because you are shy with other people?		
4	Is drinking affecting your reputation?		
5	Have you ever felt remorse after drinking?		
6	Have you got into financial difficulties as a result of drinking?		
7	Do you turn to lower companions and an inferior environment when drinking?		
8	Does your drinking make you careless of your family's welfare?		
9	Has your ambition decreased since drinking?		
10	Do you crave a drink at a definite time daily?		
11	Do you want a drink the next morning?		
12	Does drinking cause you to have difficulty sleeping?		
13	Has your efficiency decreased since drinking?		
14	Is drinking jeopardizing your job or business?		
15	Do you drink to escape from worries or trouble?		
16	Do you drink alone?		
17	Have you ever had a complete loss of memory as a result of drinking?		
18	Has your physician ever treated you for drinking?		
19	Do you drink to build up your self-confidence?		
20	Have you ever been to a hospital or institution on account of drinking?		

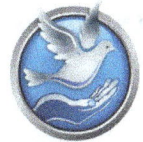

© 2024 – ANMOL JEEVAN FOUNDATION – PROPRIETARY AWARENESS & TRAINING MATERIAL FOR RECOVERING DRUG / SEX / CYBER / PORN ADDICTS, ALCOHOLICS, GAMBLERS, PSYCHIATRIC ILLNESS AND PERSONALITY DISORDERS.

- IF YOU HAVE ANSWERED **YES** TO ANY OF THE QUESTIONS, THERE IS A DEFINITE WARNING THAT YOU MAY BE ALCOHOLIC.

- IF YOU HAVE ANSWERED **YES TO ANY 2**, THE CHANCES ARE THAT YOU ARE AN ALCOHOLIC.

- IF YOU HAVE ANSWERED **YES TO 3** OR MORE, YOU ARE DEFINITELY AN ALCOHOLIC.

- HOW MANY QUESTIONS DID YOU ANSWER **YES TO**? _____

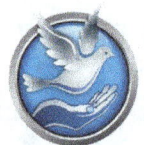 © 2024 – ANMOL JEEVAN FOUNDATION – PROPRIETARY AWARENESS & TRAINING MATERIAL FOR RECOVERING DRUG / SEX / CYBER / PORN ADDICTS, ALCOHOLICS, GAMBLERS, PSYCHIATRIC ILLNESS AND PERSONALITY DISORDERS.

HARMFUL EFFECTS AND CONSEQUENCES OF ADDICTION IN MY LIFE

A	PHYSICAL	BRIEF EXPLANATION:
	○ WEIGHT LOSS ○ SKIN TEXTURE ○ INJURIES ○ WITHDRAWAL SYMPTOMS, TREMORS, CONVULSIONS, ETC. ○ IMPAIRED LIVER FUNCTION (DUE TO DRINKING) ○ LUNGS/BREATHING PROBLEMS DUE TO SMOKING DRUGS ○ LOSS OF APPETITE ○ DIGESTIVE PROBLEMS ○ SLEEP PROBLEMS ○ EPILEPSY ○ TIREDNESS, FATIGUE ○ LETHARGY, LAZINESS ○ SEXUAL INABILITY ○ STAMINA ○ PHYSICAL STRENGTH ○ DENTAL HEALTH ○ BLOOD PRESSURE ○ IRREGULAR HEART RATE ○ ORGAN IMPAIRMENT ○ SKIN INFECTIONS	

THE ANMOL JEEVAN ACCELERATED RECOVERY & RELAPSE MANAGEMENT PROGRAM™

	○ URINARY PROBLEMS ○ RESTLESSNESS ○ SEXUALLY TRANSMITTED DISEASE ○ HYPER ACIDITY ○ INFECTIONS DUE TO CONTAMINATED NEEDLES/BLOOD ○ HAIR LICE ○ ETC.	
B	MENTAL/INTELLECTUAL	BRIEF EXPLANATION:
	○ CONFUSION ○ DELUSIONS, HALLUCINATIONS ○ MEMORY IMPAIRMENT ○ LACK OF CONCENTRATION, FOCUS ○ ATTENTION DEFICIT ○ COGNITIVE DYSFUNCTION ○ BOREDOM ○ DELAYED GRATIFICATION ○ GENERAL LOSS OF INTEREST IN ACTIVITIES ○ CONSTANT THINKING / OVER THINKING / REPETITIVE THINKING	

		BRIEF EXPLANATION:
	○ MIND-BODY COORDINATION PROBLEMS ○ BAD JUDGEMENT ○ BLANKNESS ○ ADDICTION RELATED MENTAL DISORDERS ○ ETC.	

C	EMOTIONAL	BRIEF EXPLANATION:
	○ ANGER, AGGRESSION ○ FEAR, ANXIETY, INSECURITY, PARANOIA ○ DEPRESSION, SADNESS ○ MOOD SWINGS ○ LONELINESS ○ HATRED, RESENTMENT ○ SELF-PITY ○ IMPULSIVENESS ○ IMPATIENCE ○ INTOLERANCE ○ STRESS ○ GUILT, REMORSE ○ SHAME, ASHAMED OF BODY ○ FRUSTRATION, IRRITATION ○ SUICIDAL THOUGHTS ○ HOPELESSNESS	

D	SOCIAL	BRIEF EXPLANATION:
	○ SOCIAL ANXIETY ○ INABILITY TO BEGIN OR SUSTAIN CONVERSATIONS ○ SHYNESS ○ FALSE PRIDE, EGO ○ DYSFUNCTIONAL INTERPERSONAL RELATIONSHIPS ○ BARGAINING, BLACKMAILING ○ DEMANDING, EXPECTATION ○ DEPENDENCE ○ DOMINANCE ○ STUBBORN ○ ISOLATION ○ NON-SUPPORTIVE ○ NON-COOPERATIVE ○ DISOBEDIENT ○ CO-DEPENDENCY ○ EXTRA-MARITAL RELATIONSHIPS ○ DISLOYAL ○ ILLICIT RELATIONSHIPS ○ UNWELCOME IN FAMILY DECISION MAKING PROCESS ○ PAID SEXUAL RELATIONSHIPS ○ ANTISOCIAL BEHAVIOUR ○ POOR HELP-SEEKING BEHAVIOUR	

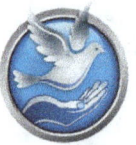

	○ SOCIAL REJECTION ○ POOR PARENTING ○ MUTUAL DISTRUST ○ CONTROL ISSUES	
E	FINANCIAL	BRIEF EXPLANATION:
	○ RECKLESS BORROWING, LOANS/DEBTS ○ RECKLESS SPENDING, GRANDIOSE ○ SPENDING MONEY KEPT FOR OTHER THINGS ON ALCOHOL/DRUGS ○ NO SAVINGS ○ LOSSES ○ NO CREDITWORTHINESS ○ LOSS OF PROPERTY, VALUABLES ○ FINANCIAL DEPENDENCE ○ RISK OF NOT GETTING YOUR FINANCIAL RIGHTS	
F	LEGAL	BRIEF EXPLANATION:

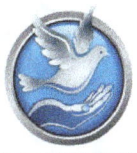

	○ ENCOUNTERS WITH LAW ENFORCEMENT AUTHORITIES ○ JAILS, LOCK-UPS ○ DIVORCE ISSUES ○ PROPERTY ISSUES ○ CIVIL CASES, FINANCIAL CRIMES ○ DRUNKEN DRIVING ○ ACCIDENT CASES ○ DRUG-RELATED LEGAL PROBLEMS ○ DOMESTIC VIOLENCE ○ PUBLIC NUISANCE ○ PETTY CRIMES ○ RESTRAINING ORDERS ○ FINES	
G	JOB/CAREER/EDUCATION	BRIEF EXPLANATION:
	○ SCHOOL COLLEGE DROPOUT ○ ABSENTEEISM ○ POOR SCHOOL/COLLEGE GRADES ○ LOSS OF JOBS ○ MISSED OPPORTUNITIES ○ UN-EMPLOYABILITY ○ INCONSISTENT ○ LACK OF FOCUS, CONCENTRATION	

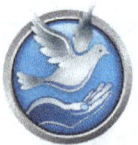

© 2024 – ANMOL JEEVAN FOUNDATION – PROPRIETARY AWARENESS & TRAINING MATERIAL FOR RECOVERING DRUG / SEX / CYBER / PORN ADDICTS, ALCOHOLICS, GAMBLERS, PSYCHIATRIC ILLNESS AND PERSONALITY DISORDERS.

	○ INABILITY TO COMPLETE ASSIGNMENTS, PROJECTS, ETC. ○ INDISCIPLINE, IRRESPONSIBLE ○ DISPUTES WITH MANAGEMENT ○ PROBLEMS WITH COLLEAGUES ○ LOSS OF AMBITION, DEGRADATION OF AMBITION ○ INABILITY TO SUSTAIN A JOB ○ LOSS OF PRODUCTIVITY	
H	SPIRITUAL	BRIEF EXPLANATION:
	○ SELF-CENTRED ○ JEALOUSY ○ MANIPULATION ○ THREATENING ○ INSENSITIVITY ○ SECRETIVE ○ DISHONESTY ○ CLOSE-MINDEDNESS ○ GREEDY ○ INCONSIDERATE ○ JUDGEMENTAL ○ PESSIMISTIC ○ DEFEATIST ○ STEALING ○ LYING	

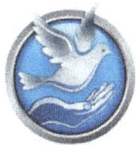

○ DECEITFULNESS ○ RUDE ○ UNFAIR ○ CRITICISM ○ BLAMING OTHERS	

	CONCLUSIONS	YES	NO
1	DO YOU ADMIT THAT YOU HAVE A DISEASE OF ALCOHOLISM / ADDICTION?		
2	DO YOU AGREE THAT YOU CAN NO LONGER DRINK/USE IN CONTROL?		
3	DO YOU NOW ACCEPT THAT YOU CAN NEVER DRINK/USE DRUGS?		
4	HAVE YOU UNDERSTOOD THAT IF YOU DRINK/USE DRUGS NOW, YOUR SITUATION COULD WORSEN?		
5	HAVE YOU REALIZED THAT ALCOHOLISM/ADDICTION HAS BEEN A PROGRESSIVELY WORSENING CONDITION IN YOUR LIFE?		
6	DO YOU BELIEVE THAT YOU HAVE PAID A HIGH PRICE IN YOUR ALCOHOLISM/ADDICTION?		
7	HAS IT OCCURRED TO YOU THAT THE CONSEQUENCES THAT YOU ARE FACING TODAY ON ACCOUNT OF ALCOHOLISM/ADDICTION ARE VERY SERIOUS?		
8	DO YOU REALIZE THAT YOU DID NOT PLAN TO REACH THIS PAINFUL STATE IN YOUR LIFE?		
9	DID YOU EVER TELL YOURSELF "I'M NOT THAT BAD"?		

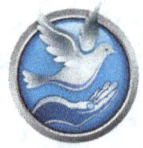

10	ARE YOU TROUBLED BY THE FACT THAT YOU CAN NEVER DRINK/USE WITHOUT CONSEQUENCES AGAIN?		
11	DO YOU THINK THAT "MAYBE", YOU DON'T HAVE THIS DISEASE AND THAT YOU WILL BE ABLE TO DRINK/USE DRUGS OCCASIONALLY?		
12	DO YOU PLAN TO DRINK/USE DRUGS SOMETIME IN THE FUTURE JUST TO FIND OUT WHETHER OR NOT YOU HAVE THE "PHYSICAL ALLERGY / CRAVING"?		
13	DO YOU THINK THAT IT WILL BE DIFFICULT FOR YOU TO LIVE WITHOUT "DRINKING/USING DRUGS" ANYMORE?		
14	DO YOU GET THE THOUGHT OF DRINKING/USING "JUST ONE TIME"?		
15	DO YOU FEEL EMPTY WITHOUT DRINKING/USING DRUGS?		

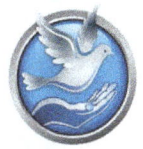 © 2024 – ANMOL JEEVAN FOUNDATION – PROPRIETARY AWARENESS & TRAINING MATERIAL FOR RECOVERING DRUG / SEX / CYBER / PORN ADDICTS, ALCOHOLICS, GAMBLERS, PSYCHIATRIC ILLNESS AND PERSONALITY DISORDERS.

WHAT IS THE NATURE OF MY MENTAL OBSESSION, PHYSICAL COMPULSION AND SPIRITUAL BANKRUPTCY?

MENTAL OBSESSION	EXAMPLES:
○ THE INSANE DESIRE FOR ALCOHOL/DRUG OF YOUR CHOICE. ○ THE MENTAL PREOCCUPATION WITH ALCOHOL/DRUG OF CHOICE – CONTINUOUSLY THINKING OF ALCOHOL / DRUG OF CHOICE. ○ BECOMING DESPERATE OR IMPATIENT WHEN YOU DON'T GET THE OPPORTUNITY TO GO AND DRINK/USE DRUGS. ○ SELECTIVELY REMEMBERING ONLY THE PLEASURE GIVEN BY ALCOHOL/DRUG OF CHOICE AND IGNORING THE PAIN AND TROUBLE CAUSED BY IT. ○ NOT AT ALL FEELING GOOD WHEN NOT UNDER THE INFLUENCE OF ALCOHOL/DRUG OF CHOICE AND BELIEVING THAT ONLY ALCOHOL/DRUG OF CHOICE CAN MAKE YOU FEEL BETTER. ○ FEEL ABNORMAL WITHOUT DRINKING/USING DRUGS. ○ UNABLE TO LET GO OF THE THOUGHT OF DRINKING/USING DRUGS.	

○ SUBSTITUTING ONE DRUG FOR ANOTHER, TRYING OUT VARIOUS DRINKING METHODS, USING A COMBINATION OF DRUGS AND ALCOHOL TO GET MORE AND MORE HIGH. ○ DESPERATELY WANTING ALCOHOL/DRUG OF CHOICE HERE & NOW. ○ FEAR OF NOT GETTING ALCOHOL/DRUG OF CHOICE. ○ EVERY TIME YOU STOP … YOU START AGAIN. ○ BELIEVING THAT YOU CAN DRINK/USE IN CONTROL.	

PHYSICAL ALLERGY/PHYSICAL CRAVING/COMPULSION	EXAMPLES:
○ NOT AT ALL SATISFIED WITH A LITTLE ALCOHOL/DRUG OF CHOICE – WANTING MORE AND MORE. ○ CANNOT SAY "NO" TO ALCOHOL/DRUGS. ○ ONCE HAVING CONSUMED ALCOHOL/DRUG OF CHOICE, YOU CANNOT CONTROL IT ANYMORE. THE DRINKING/USING CYCLE CONTINUES FOR DAYS, WEEKS, MONTHS AND EVEN YEARS.	

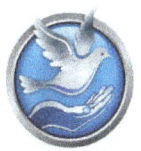

○ CONTINUE TO DRINK/USE DRUGS IN-SPITE OF FAMILY PRESSURE, PRESSURE FROM WORK, FRIENDS, ETC. ○ UNABLE TO STOP DESPITE HEALTH PROBLEMS, MONEY PROBLEMS, RELATIONSHIP PROBLEMS, CAREER/JOB PROBLEMS, ETC. ○ NOT ABLE TO KEEP UP PROMISES TO STOP. ○ USING ALCOHOL/DRUG OF CHOICE UNTIL BLACKOUTS / OVERDOSE. ○ FIND IT DIFFICULT TO KEEP ALCOHOL/DRUG OF CHOICE FOR THE NEXT DAY OR NEXT FEW DAYS. (UNABLE TO DRINK/USE IN CONTROL) ○ DRINKING/USING ROUND-THE-CLOCK. ○ THE MORE YOU DRINK/USE DRUGS, THE MORE YOU WANT.	

SPIRITUAL BANKRUPTCY / SPIRITUAL DEGENERATION	EXAMPLES:
○ INABILITY TO DIFFERENTIATE BETWEEN RIGHT AND WRONG. ○ BECOMING EXTREMELY SELF-CENTRED AND SELF-OBSESSED.	

- ◯ NOT CARING FOR OTHERS' FEELINGS.
- ◯ NOT FULFILLING RESPONSIBILITIES.
- ◯ LYING, CHEATING, CONNING.
- ◯ BORROWING, BEGGING, STEALING.
- ◯ DO THINGS THAT GO AGAINST YOUR VALUES.
- ◯ ANTI-SOCIAL, DEVIANT BEHAVIOUR, REBELLIOUS BEHAVIOUR.
- ◯ ISOLATION FROM OTHERS.
- ◯ BLAMING, PLAYING VICTIM.
- ◯ DISTRUST OF OTHERS, SUSPICIOUSNESS.
- ◯ SECRETIVENESS
- ◯ DEFIANCE
- ◯ NOT ACCEPTING YOUR OWN MISTAKES.
- ◯ VIOLENCE, AGGRESSION, ANGER, ABUSIVENESS.
- ◯ COMPLAINING, CRITICISMS.
- ◯ RUNNING AWAY FROM PROBLEMS / PEOPLE / PLACES.
- ◯ CAUSING HURT TO OTHERS.
- ◯ UNREPENTANT, JUSTIFYING.
- ◯ BITTERNESS AND HATRED TOWARDS THOSE WHO DISAPPROVE OF YOUR ALCOHOL/DRUG USE.
- ◯ SELF-DESTRUCTION
- ◯ INABILITY TO GIVE AND RECEIVE LOVE.

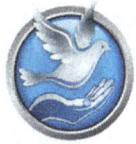

○ INABILITY TO TAKE POSITIVE ACTION. ○ OTHER:	

COMMENTS:

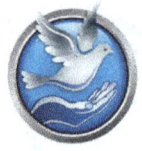 © 2024 – ANMOL JEEVAN FOUNDATION – PROPRIETARY AWARENESS & TRAINING MATERIAL FOR RECOVERING DRUG / SEX / CYBER / PORN ADDICTS, ALCOHOLICS, GAMBLERS, PSYCHIATRIC ILLNESS AND PERSONALITY DISORDERS.

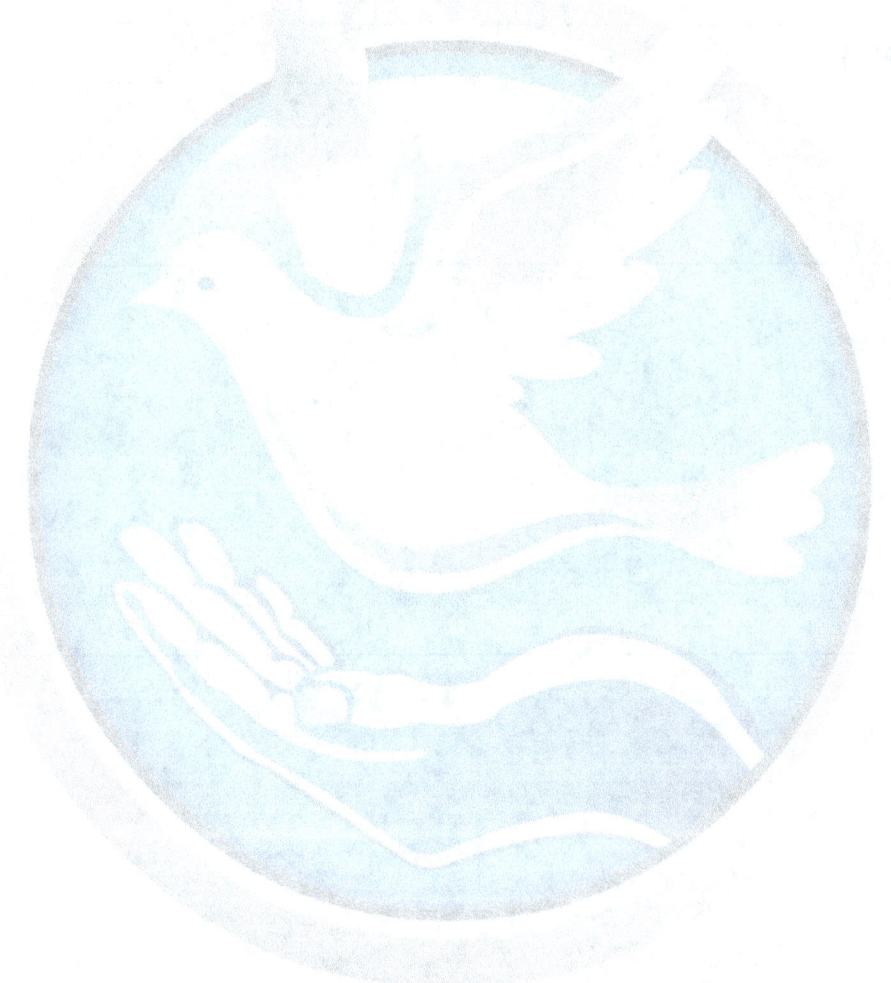

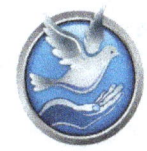 © 2024 – ANMOL JEEVAN FOUNDATION – PROPRIETARY AWARENESS & TRAINING MATERIAL FOR RECOVERING DRUG / SEX / CYBER / PORN ADDICTS, ALCOHOLICS, GAMBLERS, PSYCHIATRIC ILLNESS AND PERSONALITY DISORDERS.

AUTOBIOGRAPHY

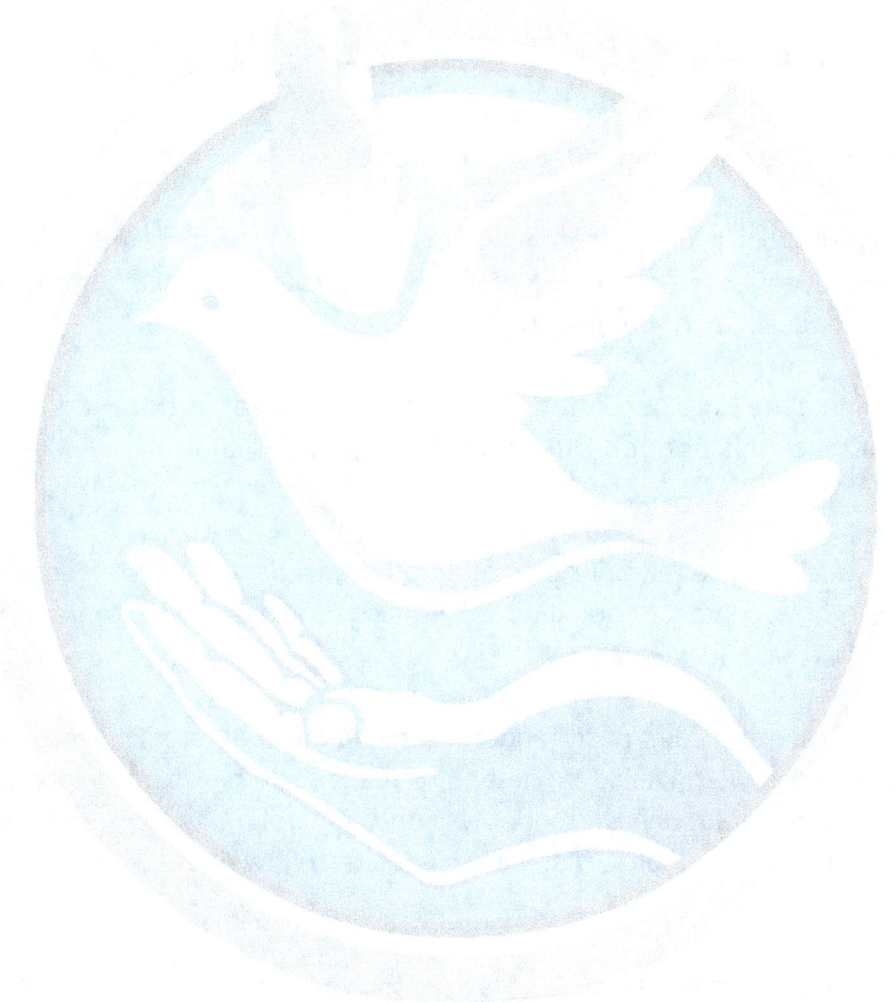

© 2024 – ANMOL JEEVAN FOUNDATION – PROPRIETARY AWARENESS & TRAINING MATERIAL FOR RECOVERING DRUG / SEX / CYBER / PORN ADDICTS, ALCOHOLICS, GAMBLERS, PSYCHIATRIC ILLNESS AND PERSONALITY DISORDERS.

STEP ONE –
WE ADMITTED THAT WE WERE POWERLESS OVER OUR ADDICTION AND THAT OUR LIVES HAD BECOME UNMANAGEABLE

The **First Step** is the beginning of recovery process.

We've been around awhile, abstinent form drugs, but we've discovered that our disease has become active in some other area of our lives, forcing us to face our powerlessness and the unmanageability of our lives once again.

Some of us find a measure of comfort in realizing that a disease, not a moral failing, has caused us to reach this bottom. Others don't really care what the cause has been—we just want out!

Our hope is to internalize the principles of Step One, to deepen our surrender, to make the principles of acceptance, humility, willingness, honesty, and open-mindedness a fundamental part of who we are.

First, we must arrive at a point of surrender. There are many different ways to do this. For some of us, the road we travelled on getting to the First Step was more than enough to convince us that unconditional surrender was our only option. Only in working the First Step do we truly come to realize that we are addicts, that we have hit bottom, and that we must surrender.

If we've been clean awhile and our First Step is about our powerlessness over some other behavior that's made our lives unmanageable, we need to find a way to stop the behavior so that our surrender isn't clouded by continued acting out.

The Disease of Addiction

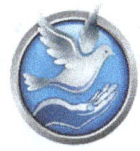

© 2024 – ANMOL JEEVAN FOUNDATION – PROPRIETARY AWARENESS & TRAINING MATERIAL FOR RECOVERING DRUG / SEX / CYBER / PORN ADDICTS, ALCOHOLICS, GAMBLERS, PSYCHIATRIC ILLNESS AND PERSONALITY DISORDERS.

What makes us addicts is the disease of abdication—not the drugs/alcohol, not our behavior, but our disease. There is something within us that makes us unable to control our use of drugs/alcohol. This same "something" also makes us prone to obsession and compulsion in other areas of our lives. How can we tell when our disease is active? When we become trapped in obsessive, compulsive, self-centered routines, endless loops that lead nowhere but to physical, mental, spiritual, and emotional decay.

When a thought occurs to me, do I immediately act on it without considering the consequences? In what other ways do I behave compulsively?

जेव्हा माझ्या मनात एखादा विचार येतो, तेव्हा परिणामांचा विचार न करता मी लगेच त्यावर कृती करतो का? मी इतर कोणत्या मार्गांनी सक्तीने वागतो?

जब मेरे मन में कोई विचार आता है, तो क्या मैं परिणामों पर विचार किए बिना तुरंत उस पर कार्य करता हूं? मैं और किन तरीकों से बाध्यकारी ढंग से व्यवहार करता हूँ?

જ્યારે મને કોઈ વિચાર આવે છે, ત્યારે શું હું પરિણામને ધ્યાનમાં લીધા વિના તરત જ તેના પર કાર્ય કરું છું? અન્ય કઈ રીતે હું અનિવાર્ય વર્તન કરું?

_____
_____
_____
_____
_____
_____
_____
_____
_____
_____
_____
_____
_____
_____

How does the self-centered part of my disease affect my life and the lives of those around me?

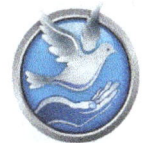

© 2024 – ANMOL JEEVAN FOUNDATION – PROPRIETARY AWARENESS & TRAINING MATERIAL FOR RECOVERING DRUG / SEX / CYBER / PORN ADDICTS, ALCOHOLICS, GAMBLERS, PSYCHIATRIC ILLNESS AND PERSONALITY DISORDERS.

माझ्या रोगाचा स्वकेंद्रित भाग माझ्या आयुष्यावर आणि माझ्या सभोवतालच्या लोकांच्या जीवनावर कसा परिणाम करतो?

मेरी बीमारी का आत्मकेंद्रित हिस्सा मेरे जीवन और मेरे आसपास के लोगों के जीवन को कैसे प्रभावित करता है?

મારા રોગનો સ્વ-કેન્દ્રિત ભાગ મારા જીવન અને મારી આસપાસના લોકોના જીવનને કેવી રીતે અસર કરે છે?

_____
_____
_____
_____
_____
_____
_____
_____
_____
_____
_____
_____
_____
_____
_____
_____
_____
_____
_____
_____
_____
_____
_____
_____
_____

How has my disease affected me physically? Mentally? Spiritually? Emotionally?

माझ्या आजाराने माझ्यावर शारीरिकरित्या कसा परिणाम केला आहे? मानसिकदृष्ट्या? आध्यात्मिकदृष्ट्या? भावनिकदृष्ट्या?

मेरी बीमारी ने मुझे शारीरिक रूप से कैसे प्रभावित किया है? मानसिक रूप से? आध्यात्मिक रूप से? भावनात्मक रूप से?

મારી બીમારીએ મને શારીરિક રીતે કેવી અસર કરી છે? માનસિક રીતે? આધ્યાત્મિક રીતે? ભાવનાત્મક રીતે?

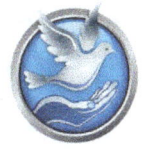

© 2024 – ANMOL JEEVAN FOUNDATION – PROPRIETARY AWARENESS & TRAINING MATERIAL FOR RECOVERING DRUG / SEX / CYBER / PORN ADDICTS, ALCOHOLICS, GAMBLERS, PSYCHIATRIC ILLNESS AND PERSONALITY DISORDERS.

Denial

Denial is the part of our disease that tells us we don't have a disease. When we are in denial, we are unable to see the reality of our addiction. We minimize its effect. We blame others, citing the too-high expectations of families, friends, and employers. We compare ourselves with other addicts whose addiction seems "worse" than our own. We may blame one particular drug/alcohol. If we have been abstinent from drugs/alcohol for some time, we might compare the current manifestation of our addiction with our drug/alcohol use, rationalizing that nothing we do today could possibly be as bad as that was! One of the easiest ways to tell that we are in denial is when we find ourselves giving plausible but untrue reasons for our behavior.

How have I blamed other people for my behavior? How have I been dishonest about my actions, behavior and the consequences?

माझ्या वर्तनासाठी मी इतर लोकांना दोष कसा दिला? मी माझ्या कृती, वर्तन आणि परिणामांबद्दल अप्रामाणिक कसे झालो?

मैंने अपने व्यवहार के लिए दूसरे लोगों को कैसे दोषी ठहराया है? मैं अपने कार्यों, व्यवहार और परिणामों के बारे में कैसे बेईमान रहा हूँ?

મારા વર્તન માટે મેં અન્ય લોકોને કેવી રીતે દોષી ઠેરવ્યા છે? હું મારા કાર્યો, વર્તન અને પરિણામો વિશે કેવી રીતે અપ્રમાણિક રહ્યો છું?

How have I compared my addiction with others' addictions? Have I justified my addiction by comparing it to other people? Have I told myself, or others that I am still in control of my addiction?

मी माझ्या व्यसनाची इतरांच्या व्यसनांशी तुलना कशी केली आहे? मी माझ्या व्यसनाची इतर लोकांशी तुलना करून त्याचे समर्थन केले आहे का? मी स्वतःला किंवा इतरांना सांगितले आहे की मी अजूनही माझ्या व्यसनावर नियंत्रण ठेवत आहे?

मैंने अपनी लत की तुलना दूसरों के व्यसनों से कैसे की है? क्या मैंने अन्य लोगों से इसकी तुलना करके अपनी लत को सही ठहराया है? क्या मैंने अपने आप को, या दूसरों को बताया है कि मैं अभी भी अपनी लत पर नियंत्रण में हूँ?

મેં મારા વ્યસનને અન્યના વ્યસન સાથે કેવી રીતે સરખાવ્યું છે? શું મેં મારા વ્યસનને અન્ય લોકો સાથે સરખાવીને યોગ્ય ઠેરવ્યું છે? શું મેં મારી જાતને અથવા અન્યને કહ્યું છે કે હું હજુ પણ મારા વ્યસન પર નિયંત્રણમાં છું?

Hitting bottom: Despair and Isolation

Our addiction finally brings us to a place where we can no longer deny the nature of our problem. All the lies, all the rationalizations, all the illusions fall away as we stand face-to-face with what our lives have become. We realize we've been living without hope. We find we've become friendless or so completely disconnected that our relationships are a sham, a parody of love and intimacy. Though it may seem that all is lost when we find ourselves in this state, the truth is that we must pass through this place before we can embark upon our journey of recovery.

When did I realize that my addiction has gone beyond my control? What are the reasons that I am being forced into rehabilitation or recovery?

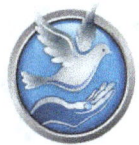

माझे व्यसन माझ्या नियंत्रणाबाहेर गेले आहे हे मला कधी कळले? मला पुनर्वसन किंवा पुनर्प्राप्तीसाठी भाग पाडले जात असल्याची कोणती कारणे आहेत?

मुझे कब एहसास हुआ कि मेरी लत मेरे नियंत्रण से बाहर हो गई है? क्या कारण हैं कि मुझे पुनर्वास या पुनर्प्राप्ति के लिए मजबूर किया जा रहा है?

મને ક્યારે ખ્યાલ આવ્યો કે મારું વ્યસન મારા નિયંત્રણની બહાર ગયું છે? કયા કારણો છે કે મને પુનર્વસન અથવા પુનઃપ્રાપ્તિ માટે ફરજ પાડવામાં આવી રહી છે?

When I realized that my addiction is out of control, what efforts did I make to control my addiction? What was the result of the effort that I made?

माझे व्यसन नियंत्रणाबाहेर गेले आहे हे लक्षात आल्यावर मी माझ्या व्यसनावर नियंत्रण ठेवण्यासाठी कोणते प्रयत्न केले? मी केलेल्या प्रयत्नांचे फळ काय मिळाले?

जब मैंने महसूस किया कि मेरी लत नियंत्रण से बाहर हो गई है, तो मैंने अपनी लत को नियंत्रित करने के लिए क्या प्रयास किए? मैंने जो मेहनत की उसका नतीजा क्या निकला?

જ્યારે મને સમજાયું કે મારું વ્યસન નિયંત્રણની બહાર છે, ત્યારે મેં મારા વ્યસનને નિયંત્રિત કરવા માટે કયા પ્રયત્નો કર્યા? મેં કરેલા પ્રયત્નોનું શું પરિણામ આવ્યું?

Powerlessness

We are powerless when the driving force in our life if beyond our control. Our addiction certainly qualifies as such an uncontrollable, driving force. We cannot moderate or control our drug/alcohol use or other compulsive behaviors, even when they are causing

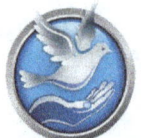

us to lose the things that matter most to us. We cannot stop, even when to continue will surely result in irreparable physical damage. We find ourselves doing things that we would never do if it weren't for our addiction, things that make us shudder with shame when we think of them. We may even decide that we don't' want to use, that we aren't going to use, and realize we are simply unable to stop when the opportunity presents itself.

We may have tried to abstain from drug use or other compulsive behaviors—perhaps with some success—for a period of time without a program, only to find that our untreated addiction eventually takes us right back to where we were before.

What is my understanding of the concept of "Powerlessness"? Over what exactly am I powerless?

"शक्तीहीनता" या संकल्पनेबद्दल माझी समज काय आहे? मी नेमका कशासाठी शक्तीहीन आहे?

"शक्तिहीनता" की अवधारणा के बारे में मेरी समझ क्या है? मैं वास्तव में किस पर शक्तिहीन हूँ?

"શક્તિહીનતા" ના ખ્યાલ વિશે મારી સમજ શું છે? હું ખરેખર શા માટે શક્તિહીન છું?

_____
_____
_____
_____
_____
_____
_____
_____
_____
_____
_____
_____
_____
_____

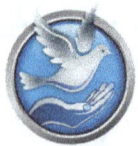

© 2024 – ANMOL JEEVAN FOUNDATION – PROPRIETARY AWARENESS & TRAINING MATERIAL FOR RECOVERING DRUG / SEX / CYBER / PORN ADDICTS, ALCOHOLICS, GAMBLERS, PSYCHIATRIC ILLNESS AND PERSONALITY DISORDERS.

What are the things I have done to protect my addiction? (Telling lies, stealing money, or committing crimes). How have I gone against my own values and beliefs to continue my addiction?

माझे व्यसन चालू ठेवण्यासाठी मी कोणत्या गोष्टी केल्या आहेत? (खोटे बोलणे, पैसे चोरणे किंवा गुन्हा करणे). माझे व्यसन चालू ठेवण्यासाठी मी माझ्या स्वतःच्या मूल्ये आणि विश्वासांच्या विरोधात कसे गेलो?

मैंने अपनी लत को जारी रखने के लिए क्या किया है? (झूठ बोलना, पैसे चुराना या कोई अपराध करना)। मैं अपनी लत को जारी रखने के लिए अपने स्वयं के मूल्यों और विश्वासों के विरुद्ध कैसे गया हूँ?

મારું વ્યસન ચાલુ રાખવા માટે મેં શું કર્યું છે? (જૂઠું બોલવું, પૈસાની ચોરી કરવી અથવા ગુનો કરવો). મારું વ્યસન ચાલુ રાખવા માટે હું મારા પોતાના મૂલ્યો અને માન્યતાઓની વિરુદ્ધ કેવી રીતે ગયો છું?

How do I manipulate (fool or deceive) other people so that I may continue my addiction in peace? How does my personality change when I become desperate in addiction - hot-tempered, selfish, cunning, dishonest or even revenge-seeking?

मी इतर लोकांना कसे हाताळू (मूर्ख किंवा फसवू) जेणेकरून मी माझे व्यसन शांततेत चालू ठेवू शकेन? जेव्हा मी व्यसनाच्या आहारी जातो तेव्हा माझे व्यक्तिमत्व कसे बदलते - उग्र स्वभावाचा, स्वार्थी, धूर्त, अप्रामाणिक किंवा अगदी बदला घेणारा?

मैं अन्य लोगों को कैसे हेरफेर (मूर्ख या धोखा) कर सकता हूं ताकि मैं शांति से अपनी लत जारी रख सकूं? जब मैं नशे की लत में हताश हो जाता हूँ - गर्म मिजाज, स्वार्थी, चालाक, बेईमान या यहाँ तक कि बदला लेने वाला हो जाता है तो मेरा व्यक्तित्व कैसे बदल जाता है?

હું અન્ય લોકોને કેવી રીતે ચાલાકી (મૂર્ખ અથવા છેતરવું) કરી શકું જેથી હું મારું વ્યસન શાંતિથી ચાલુ રાખી શકું? જ્યારે હું વ્યસનમાં ભયાવહ બની જાઉં ત્યારે મારું વ્યક્તિત્વ કેવી રીતે બદલાય છે - ગરમ સ્વભાવનો, સ્વાર્થી, ધડાયેલું, અપ્રમાણિક અથવા તો બદલો લેવાની ઇચ્છા?

The Principle of Humility, so central to the First Step, is expressed most purely in our surrender. Humility is most easily identified as an acceptance of who we truly are — neither worse nor better than we believed we were when we were using, just human.

To practice **The Principle of Acceptance**, we must do more than merely admit that we're addicts. When we accept our addiction, we feel a profound inner change that is underscored by a rising sense of hope. We also begin to feel a sense of peace. We come to terms with our addiction, with our recovery, and with the meaning those two realities will come to have in our lives. We don't dread a future of meeting attendance, sponsor contact, and step work; instead, we begin to see recovery as a precious gift, and the work connected with it as no more trouble than other routines of life.

Very clearly, I have not been humble in my life. Where do I need humility in my life? How am I prepared to practice the principle of humility in my life?

अगदी स्पष्टपणे, मी माझ्या आयुष्यात नम्र झालो नाही. मला माझ्या आयुष्यात नम्रतेची गरज कुठे आहे? मी माझ्या जीवनात नम्रतेच्या तत्त्वाचे पालन करण्यास कसे तयार आहे?

बहुत स्पष्ट रूप से, मैं अपने जीवन में विनम्र नहीं रहा हूँ. मुझे अपने जीवन में विनम्रता की आवश्यकता कहाँ है? मैं अपने जीवन में विनम्रता के सिद्धांत का अभ्यास करने के लिए कैसे तैयार हूँ?

ખૂબ જ સ્પષ્ટપણે, હું મારા જીવનમાં નમ્ર રહ્યો નથી. મારે મારા જીવનમાં નમ્રતાની ક્યાં જરૂર છે? હું મારા જીવનમાં નમ્રતાના સિદ્ધાંતનો અભ્યાસ કરવા કેવી રીતે તૈયાર છું?

How am I coming to terms with the fact that "I am an addict"? How important is self-acceptance for staying away from drugs, alcohol, sex or gambling?

"मी व्यसनी आहे" या वस्तुस्थितीशी मी कसे जुळत आहे? ड्रग्ज, अल्कोहोल, सेक्स किंवा जुगार यापासून दूर राहण्यासाठी स्व-स्वीकृती किती महत्त्वाची आहे?

मैं इस तथ्य को कैसे स्वीकार कर सकता हूँ कि "मैं एक व्यसनी हूँ"? ड्रग्स, शराब, सेक्स या जुए से दूर रहने के लिए आत्म-स्वीकृति कितनी महत्वपूर्ण है?

"હું વ્યસની છું" એ હકીકત સાથે હું કેવી રીતે આવી રહ્યો છું? ડ્રગ્સ, આલ્કોહોલ, સેક્સ અથવા જુગારથી દૂર રહેવા માટે સ્વ-સ્વીકૃતિ કેટલી મહત્વપૂર્ણ છે?

© 2024 – ANMOL JEEVAN FOUNDATION – PROPRIETARY AWARENESS & TRAINING MATERIAL FOR RECOVERING DRUG / SEX / CYBER / PORN ADDICTS, ALCOHOLICS, GAMBLERS, PSYCHIATRIC ILLNESS AND PERSONALITY DISORDERS.

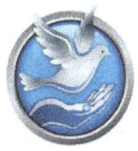

© 2024 – ANMOL JEEVAN FOUNDATION – PROPRIETARY AWARENESS & TRAINING MATERIAL FOR RECOVERING DRUG / SEX / CYBER / PORN ADDICTS, ALCOHOLICS, GAMBLERS, PSYCHIATRIC ILLNESS AND PERSONALITY DISORDERS.

STEP ONE TEST

Sr.	Questions	True	False
1	Addiction is entirely physical (of the body).		
2	Some people are born with a physical condition that puts them in high risk of becoming addicted.		
3	Addiction is influenced by social environment.		
4	Psychological pain is the primary cause of addiction.		
5	Addicted people use the addictive substance to feel normal.		
6	There is evidence that addiction is hereditary.		
7	The early stage of addiction is characterized by progressive loss of control.		
8	The chronic stage of addiction is characterized by increasing tolerance.		
9	Increased tolerance protects you from addiction.		
10	The pain of using an addictive chemical is always because of withdrawal.		
11	Rationalization is deceiving oneself about the reasons for using an addictive drug.		
12	Total abstinence is necessary to recovery from chemical addiction.		
13	Recovery is easier when you substitute a safer mood-altering drug for your drug of choice for the first few months of recovery.		
14	A common method of detoxification is administering a substitute drug.		
15	Education about addiction is essential to recovery.		
16	The best way to manage long-term withdrawal symptoms is by ignoring them and focusing on the pleasant aspects of recovery.		
17	All stages of addiction are characterized by denial.		
18	In order to recover, all stress must be eliminated from your life.		
19	Substitute addictions help people maintain abstinence from alcohol/drugs.		

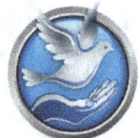

© 2024 – ANMOL JEEVAN FOUNDATION – PROPRIETARY AWARENESS & TRAINING MATERIAL FOR RECOVERING DRUG / SEX / CYBER / PORN ADDICTS, ALCOHOLICS, GAMBLERS, PSYCHIATRIC ILLNESS AND PERSONALITY DISORDERS.

20	Anger in the final stage of the relapse syndrome is often the result of the inability to control one's actions.		

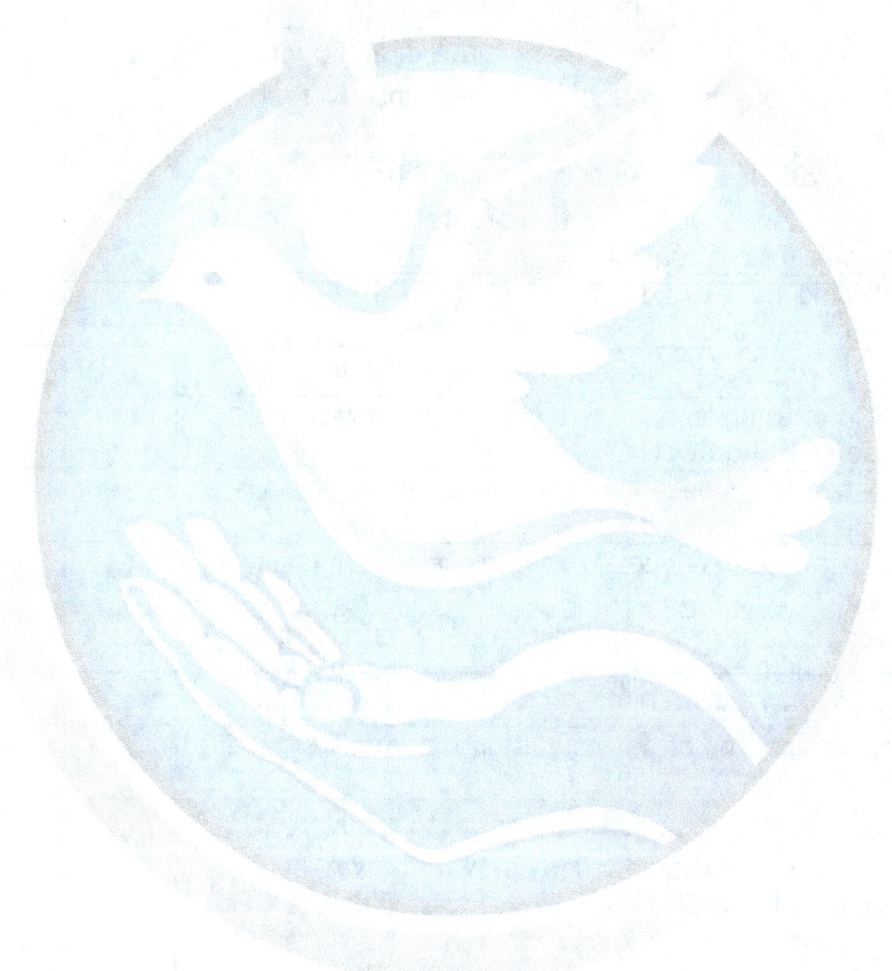

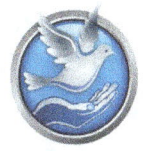

© 2024 – ANMOL JEEVAN FOUNDATION – PROPRIETARY AWARENESS & TRAINING MATERIAL FOR RECOVERING DRUG / SEX / CYBER / PORN ADDICTS, ALCOHOLICS, GAMBLERS, PSYCHIATRIC ILLNESS AND PERSONALITY DISORDERS.

STEP TWO –

WE CAME TO BELIEVE THAT A POWER GREATER THAN OURSELVES COULD RESTORE US TO SANITY

Step One strips us of our illusions about addiction; Step Two gives us hope for recovery. The pain and insanity with which we have been living are unnecessary, says Step Two. They can be relieved.

The **Second Step** fills the void we feel when we've finished Step One. As we approach Step Two, we begin to consider that maybe, just maybe, there's a Power greater than ourselves—a Power capable of healing our hurt, calming our confusion, and restoring our sanity.

From acknowledging our powerlessness to admitting our "insanity" seemed an awfully large leap. We read the Basic Text and found that our insanity was defined there as "repeating the same mistakes and expecting different results." After all, how many times had we tried to get away with something we had *never* gotten away with before, each time telling ourselves, "It will be different this time?" Now, that's insane!

Some of us resisted this step because we thought it required us to be religious. There is nothing, absolutely nothing, in the NA/AA program that requires a member to be religious. This is a spiritual, not religious, program.

The beauty of the Second Step is revealed when we begin to think about what our Higher Power can be. We are encouraged to choose a Power that is loving, caring, and—most importantly—able to restore us to sanity. The Second Step does not say, "We came to believe in a Power greater than ourselves." It says, "We came to believe that a Power greater than ourselves could restore us to sanity." The emphasis is not on who or what this Power is, but on what this Power can do for us. The group itself certainly qualifies as a Power greater than us.

So do the spiritual principles contained in the Twelve Steps. And, of course, so does the understanding any one of our individual members has of a Higher Power.

Hope

Every time we followed what we'd thought would be a path out of our addiction—medicine, religion, or psychiatry, for instance—we found they only took us so far; none of these was sufficient for us. As we ran out of options and exhausted our resources, we wondered if we'd ever find a solution to our dilemma, if there was anything in the world that worked.

However, something remarkable occurred to us as we sat in our first few meetings. There were other addicts there who had used drugs/alcohol just as we had, addicts who were now clean. We believed in them. We knew we could trust them.

It was when we realized that these other members—addicts like us—were staying clean and finding freedom that most of us first experienced the feeling of hope. We may have been listening to someone share a story just like our own.

Our hope is renewed throughout our recovery. Each time something new is revealed to us about our disease, the pain of that realization is accompanied by a surge of hope. No matter how painful the process of demolishing our denial may be, something else is being restored in its place within us. Even if we don't feel like we believe in anything, we do believe in the program. We believe that we can be restored to sanity, even in the most hopeless times, even in our sickest areas.

Insanity

If we have any doubts about the need for a renewal of sanity in our lives, we're going to have trouble with this step. Reviewing our First Step should help us if we have doubts. Now is the time to take a good look at our insanity. Insanity is a loss of our perspective and our sense of proportion. For example, we may think that our personal problems are more important than anyone else's; in fact, we may not even be able to consider other people's needs at all. Small problems become major catastrophes. Our lives get out of

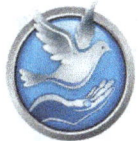

balance. Some obvious examples of insane thinking are the belief that we can stay clean on our own, or the belief that using drugs/alcohol was our only problem and that everything is fine now just because we're clean. In NA/AA, insanity is often described as the belief that we can take something outside ourselves—drugs, power, sex, food—to fix what's wrong inside ourselves: our feelings.

About what exactly do I have "Hope" today? What has changed in me, Why was I hopeless before?

आज माझ्याकडे "आशा" नक्की कशाबद्दल आहे? माझ्यात काय बदल झाला आहे, मी आधी हताश का होतो?

आज मेरे पास वास्तव में "आशा" क्या है? क्या बदला है मुझमें, मैं पहले क्यों मायूस था?

આજે મારી પાસે "હોપ" બરાબર શેના વિશે છે? મારામાં શું બદલાયું છે, પહેલા હું કેમ નિરાશ હતો?

_____
_____
_____
_____
_____
_____
_____
_____
_____
_____
_____
_____
_____
_____
_____
_____
_____

What made me think that I could "Control" my use of drugs, drinking alcohol, obsessive sex, or compulsive gambling? How did I try to "Control" myself - What efforts did I make?

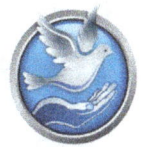

© 2024 – ANMOL JEEVAN FOUNDATION – PROPRIETARY AWARENESS & TRAINING MATERIAL FOR RECOVERING DRUG / SEX / CYBER / PORN ADDICTS, ALCOHOLICS, GAMBLERS, PSYCHIATRIC ILLNESS AND PERSONALITY DISORDERS.

मी माझ्या ड्रग्जचा वापर, दारू पिणे, वेड लावणारा सेक्स किंवा सक्तीचा जुगार खेळणे "नियंत्रित" करू शकेन असे मला कशामुळे वाटले? मी स्वतःला "नियंत्रण" करण्याचा प्रयत्न कसा केला - मी कोणते प्रयत्न केले?

किस बात ने मुझे यह सोचने पर मजबूर किया कि मैं अपने नशीली दवाओं के उपयोग, शराब पीने, जुनूनी सेक्स, या बाध्यकारी जुए को "नियंत्रित" कर सकता हूँ? मैंने स्वयं को "नियंत्रित" करने का प्रयास कैसे किया - मैंने क्या प्रयास किए?

મને શું લાગે છે કે હું મારા ડ્રગ્સનો ઉપયોગ, આલ્કોહોલ પીવું, બાધ્યતા સેક્સ અથવા અનિવાર્ય જુગારનો ઉપયોગ "નિયંત્રણ" કરી શકું? મેં મારી જાતને કેવી રીતે "નિયંત્રણ" કરવાનો પ્રયાસ કર્યો - મેં કયા પ્રયત્નો કર્યા?

_____
_____
_____
_____
_____
_____
_____
_____
_____
_____
_____
_____
_____
_____
_____
_____
_____
_____
_____
_____
_____
_____

What are the "Insane" actions that I took, as a result of my addiction? What are some of the things I did that I can hardly believe? (Example: Putting myself or others in danger, verbal, physical or sexual abuse, excessive spending and piling on debt)

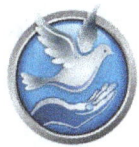

© 2024 – ANMOL JEEVAN FOUNDATION – PROPRIETARY AWARENESS & TRAINING MATERIAL FOR RECOVERING DRUG / SEX / CYBER / PORN ADDICTS, ALCOHOLICS, GAMBLERS, PSYCHIATRIC ILLNESS AND PERSONALITY DISORDERS.

माझ्या व्यसनामुळे मी केलेल्या "वेडे" कृती काय आहेत? मी अशा कोणत्या गोष्टी केल्या आहेत ज्यावर माझा विश्वास बसत नाही? (उदाहरण: स्वतःला किंवा इतरांना धोक्यात घालणे, शाब्दिक, शारीरिक किंवा लैंगिक शोषण, जास्त खर्च आणि कर्जांचा ढीग)

मेरी लत के परिणामस्वरूप, मैंने जो "पागल" कार्य किए, वे क्या हैं? मैंने ऐसी कौन सी चीज़ें की हैं जिन पर मुझे शायद ही विश्वास हो? (उदाहरण: खुद को या दूसरों को खतरे में डालना, मौखिक, शारीरिक या यौन शोषण, अत्यधिक खर्च और कर्ज का अंबार)

મારા વ્યસનના પરિણામે મેં લીધેલી "પાગલ" ક્રિયાઓ શું છે? મેં એવી કઈ વસ્તુઓ કરી છે કે જેના પર હું ભાગ્યે જ વિશ્વાસ કરી શકું? (ઉદાહરણ: મારી જાતને અથવા અન્યને જોખમમાં મૂકવું, મૌખિક, શારીરિક અથવા જાતીય શોષણ, અતિશય ખર્ચ અને દેવું)

___

___

___

___

___

___

___

___

___

___

___

___

___

___

___

___

___

___

___

___

___

___

___

How many times did act insane, as well as impulsively? What are the hasty decisions I took, that I now regret? (Examples: Quitting my job, Taking loans, Stealing money, Giving up on ambitions and plans, Breaking up relationships or friendships).

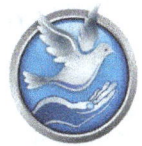

किती वेळा वेडेपणाने, तसेच आवेगपूर्ण वागले? मी घाईघाईने घेतलेले कोणते निर्णय आहेत, ज्याचा मला आता पश्चाताप होतोय? (उदाहरणे: माझी नोकरी सोडणे, कर्ज घेणे, पैसे चोरणे, महत्वाकांक्षा आणि योजना सोडणे, नातेसंबंध किंवा मैत्री तोडणे).

कितनी बार पागलपन के साथ-साथ आवेगपूर्ण व्यवहार किया? मैंने जल्दबाजी में कौन से फैसले लिए, जिनका मुझे अब पछतावा है? (उदाहरण: अपनी नौकरी छोड़ना, कर्ज लेना, पैसे चुराना, महत्वाकांक्षाओं और योजनाओं को छोड़ना, रिश्तों या दोस्ती को तोड़ना)।

કેટલી વાર પાગલ, તેમજ આવેગજન્ય વર્તન કર્યું? મેં એવા કયા ઉતાવળા નિર્ણયો લીધા છે, જેનો મને હવે પસ્તાવો થાય છે? (ઉદાહરણ: મારી નોકરી છોડવી, લોન લેવી, પૈસાની ચોરી કરવી, મહત્વાકાંક્ષાઓ અને યોજનાઓ છોડી દેવી, સંબંધો અથવા મિત્રતા તોડી નાખવી).

Do I think that drinking alcohol, taking drugs, gambling or compulsive sex is my only problem(s)? What are the other issues that I have to take care of?

मला असे वाटते की दारू पिणे, ड्रग्ज घेणे, जुगार खेळणे किंवा सक्तीचे लैंगिक संबंध ही माझी एकमेव समस्या आहे? इतर कोणत्या समस्या आहेत ज्यांची मला काळजी घ्यावी लागेल?

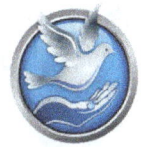

क्या मुझे लगता है कि शराब पीना, ड्रग्स लेना, जुआ खेलना या बाध्यकारी सेक्स करना ही मेरी एकमात्र समस्या है? मुझे किन अन्य मुद्दों पर ध्यान देना है?

શું મને લાગે છે કે આલ્કોહોલ પીવું, ડ્રગ્સ લેવું, જુગાર અથવા ફરજિયાત સેક્સ એ મારી એકમાત્ર સમસ્યા છે? અન્ય કયા મુદ્દાઓ છે જેની મારે કાળજી લેવી પડશે?

Despite knowing the bad outcome, why did I go ahead with my actions? What forced me to go ahead and act insane?

वाईट परिणाम माहीत असूनही मी माझ्या कृतीत का पुढे गेलो? मला पुढे जाऊन वेड्यासारखे वागण्यास कशाने भाग पाडले?

बुरे परिणाम को जानते हुए भी, मैं अपने कर्मों को आगे क्यों बढ़ाता रहा? मुझे आगे बढ़ने और पागल होने के लिए क्या मजबूर किया?

ખરાબ પરિણામ જાણવા છતાં હું મારા કાર્યોમાં કેમ આગળ વધ્યો? મને આગળ વધવા અને પાગલ વર્તન કરવા માટે શું મજબૂર કર્યું?

What have I started believing in now? How has my faith evolved as I stay away from alcohol, drugs, sex or gambling?

मी आता कशावर विश्वास ठेवायला सुरुवात केली आहे? मी दारू, ड्रग्ज, सेक्स किंवा जुगार यापासून दूर राहिल्याने माझा विश्वास कसा विकसित झाला आहे?

मैं अब किस पर विश्वास करने लगा हूं? शराब, ड्रग्स, सेक्स या जुए से दूर रहने से मेरा विश्वास कैसे विकसित हुआ है?

હું હવે શેમાં વિશ્વાસ કરવા લાગ્યો છું? હું દારૂ, ડ્રગ્સ, સેક્સ અથવા જુગારથી દૂર રહીને મારી શ્રદ્ધા કેવી રીતે વિકસિત થઈ છે?

A Power Greater than Ourselves

In this step we don't have to have a lot of specific ideas about the nature or identity of that Higher Power. The kind of understanding of a Higher Power that's most important to find in the Second Step is an understanding that can *help* us. We're not concerned here with theological elegance or doctrinal adherence—we just want something that works?

Our addiction as a negative power was, without a doubt, greater than we were. Our addiction led us down a path of insanity and caused us to act differently than we wanted to behave. We need something to combat that, something at least as powerful as our addiction.

What is my understanding of " a power greater than myself"? What can be more powerful than me?

"माझ्यापेक्षा मोठी शक्ती" बद्दल माझी समज काय आहे? माझ्यापेक्षा ताकदवान काय असू शकते?

"मुझसे बड़ी शक्ति" के बारे में मेरी समझ क्या है? मुझसे ज्यादा शक्तिशाली और क्या हो सकता है?

"મારા કરતા મોટી શક્તિ" વિશે મારી સમજ શું છે? મારાથી વધુ શક્તિશાળી શું હોઇ શકે?

How can "A Power Greater Than Myself" help me to stay away from taking drugs and drinking alcohol? How will I know that this POWER is active, and working in my life?

"माझ्यापेक्षा मोठी शक्ती" मला ड्रग्ज घेण्यापासून आणि दारू पिण्यापासून दूर राहण्यास कशी मदत करू शकते? ही शक्ती सक्रिय आहे आणि माझ्या आयुष्यात कार्यरत आहे हे मला कसे कळेल?

"खुद से बड़ी ताकत" मुझे ड्रग्स लेने और शराब पीने से दूर रहने में कैसे मदद कर सकता है? मुझे कैसे पता चलेगा कि यह शक्ति सक्रिय है, और मेरे जीवन में काम कर रही है?

ડ્રગ્સ અને આલ્કોહોલ પીવાથી દૂર રહેવા માટે "મારા કરતાં વધુ શક્તિ" મને કેવી રીતે મદદ કરી શકે? મને કેવી રીતે ખબર પડશે કે આ શક્તિ સક્રિય છે, અને મારા જીવનમાં કાર્યરત છે?

Restoration to Sanity

It Works: How and Why defines the term "restoration" as "changing to a point where addiction and its accompanying insanity are not controlling our lives." We find that just as our insanity was evident in our loss of perspective and sense of proportion, so we can see sanity in our lives when we begin developing a perspective that allows us to make better decisions. We find that we have choices about how to act. We begin to have the maturity and wisdom to slow down and consider all aspects of a situation before acting.

Most of us have no trouble identifying the sanity in our lives when we compare our drug and alcohol consumption with our early recovery, our early recovery with some time

clean, and sometime clean with long-term recovery. All of this is a process, and our need for a restoration to sanity will change over time.

When we're new in the program, being restored to sanity probably means not having to use anymore; when that happens, perhaps some of the insanity that is directly and obviously tied to our using will stop. We'll quit committing crimes to get drugs/alcohol. We'll cease putting ourselves in certain degrading situations that serve no purpose but our using.

If we've been in recovery for some time, we may find that we have no trouble believing in a Power greater than ourselves that can help us stay clean, but we may not have considered what a restoration to sanity means to us beyond staying clean.

What is my understanding of the restoration of sanity? What changes are required in my thinking and actions, for the restoration of sanity?

विवेकाच्या पुनर्स्थापनेबद्दल माझी समज काय आहे? विवेक पुनर्संचयित करण्यासाठी माझ्या विचारात आणि कृतींमध्ये कोणते बदल आवश्यक आहेत?

विवेक की बहाली के बारे में मेरी समझ क्या है? विवेक की बहाली के लिए मेरी सोच और कार्यों में क्या परिवर्तन आवश्यक हैं?

વિવેક પુનઃસ્થાપિત કરવા વિશે મારી સમજ શું છે? વિવેક પુનઃસ્થાપિત કરવા માટે, મારા વિચારો અને કાર્યોમાં કયા ફેરફારોની જરૂર છે?

_____
_____
_____
_____
_____
_____
_____
_____
_____
_____

What are my expectations from others and myself, after the restoration of sanity? Are my expectations realistic, or unrealistic?

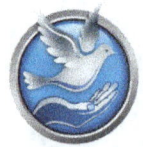 © 2024 – ANMOL JEEVAN FOUNDATION – PROPRIETARY AWARENESS & TRAINING MATERIAL FOR RECOVERING DRUG / SEX / CYBER / PORN ADDICTS, ALCOHOLICS, GAMBLERS, PSYCHIATRIC ILLNESS AND PERSONALITY DISORDERS.

विवेक पुनर्संचयित झाल्यानंतर माझ्या इतरांकडून आणि माझ्याकडून काय अपेक्षा आहेत? माझ्या अपेक्षा वास्तववादी आहेत की अवास्तव?

विवेक की बहाली के बाद, मेरी दूसरों से और स्वयं से क्या अपेक्षाएँ हैं? क्या मेरी अपेक्षाएँ यथार्थवादी हैं, या अवास्तविक हैं?

સમજદારી પુનઃસ્થાપિત કર્યા પછી, અન્ય લોકો અને મારી પાસેથી મારી અપેક્ષાઓ શું છે? મારી અપેક્ષાઓ વાસ્તવિક છે કે અવાસ્તવિક?

_____
_____
_____
_____
_____
_____
_____
_____
_____
_____
_____
_____
_____
_____
_____
_____
_____
_____
_____
_____
_____
_____

Spiritual Principles

In the Second Step, we will focus on open-mindedness, willingness, faith, trust, and humility. The principle of open-mindedness that we find in the Second Step arises from the understanding that we can't recover alone, that we need some kind of help. It continues with opening our minds to believing that help is possible for us. It doesn't matter whether we have any idea of how this Power greater than ourselves is going to help, just that we believe it's possible.

Practicing the principle of willingness in the Second Step may begin simply. At first we may just go to meetings and listen to other recovering addicts share about their experiences with this step. Then we may begin applying what we hear to our own recovery. Of course, we ask our sponsor to guide us.

How am I practicing open-mindedness today? What more changes are required in me, for retaining my sanity?

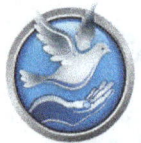

© 2024 – ANMOL JEEVAN FOUNDATION – PROPRIETARY AWARENESS & TRAINING MATERIAL FOR RECOVERING DRUG / SEX / CYBER / PORN ADDICTS, ALCOHOLICS, GAMBLERS, PSYCHIATRIC ILLNESS AND PERSONALITY DISORDERS.

मी आज खुल्या मनाचा सराव कसा करत आहे? माझा विवेक टिकवून ठेवण्यासाठी माझ्यामध्ये आणखी कोणते बदल आवश्यक आहेत?

आज मैं खुले विचारों का अभ्यास कैसे कर रहा हूँ? मेरी पवित्रता को बनाए रखने के लिए, मुझमें और कौन-से परिवर्तनों की आवश्यकता है?

આજે હું કેવી રીતે ખુલ્લા મનની પ્રેક્ટિસ કરી રહ્યો છું? મારી સમજશક્તિ જાળવી રાખવા માટે મારામાં વધુ કયા ફેરફારોની જરૂર છે?

_____
_____
_____
_____
_____
_____
_____
_____
_____
_____
_____
_____
_____
_____
_____
_____
_____
_____
_____
_____
_____
_____
_____
_____

I was unwilling to change earlier. Now that sanity has been restored what am I willing to do, that I was unwilling for before?

मी पूर्वी बदलायला तयार नव्हतो. आता बुद्धी पूर्ववत झाली आहे, मी काय करायला तयार आहे, ज्यासाठी मी पूर्वी तयार नव्हतो?

मैं पहले बदलने को तैयार नहीं था। अब जब वह विवेक बहाल हो गया है तो मैं क्या करने को तैयार हूं, जो मैं पहले नहीं करना चाहता था?

હું અગાઉ બદલવા માટે તૈયાર નહોતો. હવે વિવેક પુનઃસ્થાપિત કરવામાં આવી છે, હું શું કરવા તૈયાર છું, જે માટે હું પહેલા તૈયાર ન હતો?

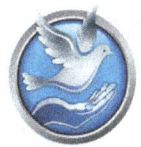

© 2024 – ANMOL JEEVAN FOUNDATION – PROPRIETARY AWARENESS & TRAINING MATERIAL FOR RECOVERING DRUG / SEX / CYBER / PORN ADDICTS, ALCOHOLICS, GAMBLERS, PSYCHIATRIC ILLNESS AND PERSONALITY DISORDERS.

STEP TWO TEST

Sr.	Questions	True	False
1	A person caught in the cycle of addiction uses his or her addiction to relieve pain caused by the addiction.		
2	Obsession is continuous thinking about the positive effects of using an addictive drug.		
3	Compulsion is the irrational urge or craving for a drug.		
4	Loss of control means addicted people cannot stop drinking/using when they intend to.		
5	Delusional thinking is a psychotic state.		
6	Counseling for addiction must be individual counseling to be effective.		
7	It is difficult to recover without a spiritual program.		
8	Living with stressful situations on a daily basis is the best way to build up your resistance to stress so that you can handle a crisis when it comes along.		
9	A triggering event for one person may not be for another person.		
10	In order to recover, you should not make any major changes for one year.		
11	How your body reacts to a stressor is not a conscious decision.		
12	Stress cycles are healthy ways of reacting to stressors.		
13	When you cannot solve a problem causing stress you can find other ways to manage stress.		
14	You should take a different time for prayer and meditation every day.		
15	A spiritual program requires membership in a church/temple/mosque		
16	To have a spiritual program you must accept the possibility that there is a power greater than yourself.		
17	Most people do not need a quiet place for meditation; it is what is going on inside that matter, not what is going on around you.		
18	Dissatisfaction with life may lead to the recovering person seeing alcohol/drug use as a way of making things better.		
19	Self-help group members are not helpful to the recovering person in the later stages of the relapse syndrome.		
20	When a person returns to addictive use denial keeps him from feeling shame or guilt.		

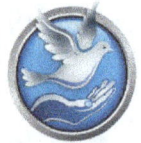

STEP THREE –
WE MADE A DECISION TO TURN OUR WILL AND OUR LIVES OVER TO THE CARE OF GOD AS WE UNDERSTOOD HIM

We do not translate our hope into action right now, it will fade away, and we'll end up right back where we started. The action we need to take is Step Three.

The central action in Step Three is a decision. The idea of making that decision may terrify us, especially when we look at what we're deciding to do in this step. Making a decision, any decision, is something most of us haven't done in a long time.

The Third Step decision may be too big to make in one leap. The Third Step is just one more piece of the path of recovery from our addiction. Making the Third Step decision doesn't necessarily mean that we must suddenly completely change everything about the way we live our lives. We don't have to be afraid that this step will do something to us that we're not ready for or won't like.

It is significant that this step suggests we turn our will and our lives over to the care of the God of our understanding. By working the Third Step, we are allowing someone or something to care for us, not control us or conduct our lives for us. This step does not suggest that we become mindless robots with no ability to live our own lives, nor does it allow those of us who find such irresponsibility attractive to indulge such an urge. Instead, we are making a simple decision to change direction, to stop rebelling at the natural and logical flow of events in our lives, to stop wearing ourselves out trying to make everything

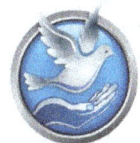

happen as if we were in charge of the world. We are accepting that a Power greater than ourselves will do a better job of caring for our will and our lives than we have.

Our concept of God will grow as we grow in our recovery. Working the Third Step will help us discover what works best for us.

Making a Decision

The decision to turn our will and lives over to the care of the God of our understanding is one we can make over and over again, daily if need be. In fact, we're likely to find that we must make this decision regularly, or risk losing our recovery because of complacency.
It is essential that we involve our hearts and spirits in this decision. Though the word "decision" sounds like something that takes place mostly in the mind, we need to do the work necessary to go beyond an intellectual understanding and internalize this choice.

Step Three is all about deciding. What are the decisions that I need to take just for today? What are some conditions that I have about making this decision? (Examples: I expect the support of others in my recovery, I will surrender everything except my finances and career, or I will stay sober only if my marriage issues are resolved).

तिसरी पायरी म्हणजे निर्णय घेणे. मला फक्त आजसाठी कोणते निर्णय घ्यावे लागतील? हा निर्णय घेताना माझ्याकडे कोणत्या काही अटी आहेत? (उदाहरणे: मला माझ्या पुनर्प्राप्तीमध्ये इतरांच्या पाठिंब्याची अपेक्षा आहे, मी माझे आर्थिक आणि करिअर सोडून सर्वकाही समर्पण करीन किंवा माझ्या लग्नाच्या समस्यांचे निराकरण झाले तरच मी शांत राहीन).

चरण तीन निर्णय लेने के बारे में है। ऐसे कौन से निर्णय हैं जो मुझे केवल आज के लिए लेने चाहिए? यह निर्णय लेने के बारे में मेरी कुछ शर्तें क्या हैं? (उदाहरण: मैं अपने सुधार में दूसरों के समर्थन की उम्मीद करता हूं, मैं अपने वित्त और करियर को छोड़कर सब कुछ आत्मसमर्पण कर दूंगा, या मैं केवल तभी शांत रहूंगा जब मेरी शादी के मुद्दों का समाधान हो जाएगा)।

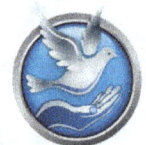

પગલું ત્રણ નક્કી કરવા વિશે છે. મારે ફક્ત આજ માટે કયા નિર્ણયો લેવાની જરૂર છે? આ નિર્ણય લેવા માટે મારી પાસે કઈ શરતો છે? (ઉદાહરણ: હું મારી પુનઃપ્રાપ્તિમાં અન્ય લોકોના સમર્થનની અપેક્ષા રાખું છું, હું મારી નાણાકીય અને કારકિર્દી સિવાય બધું જ સોંપી દઈશ, અથવા મારા લગ્નના પ્રશ્નો ઉકેલાઈ જશે તો જ હું શાંત રહીશ).

Which areas of my life are difficult to turn over? How shall I work on surrendering in these areas of my life?

माझ्या आयुष्यातील कोणते क्षेत्र बदलणे कठीण आहे? माझ्या जीवनाच्या या क्षेत्रांमध्ये मी आत्मसमर्पणावर कसे कार्य करू?

मेरे जीवन के किन क्षेत्रों को पलटना मुश्किल है? मैं अपने जीवन के इन क्षेत्रों में समर्पण पर कैसे काम करूं?

મારા જીવનના કયા ક્ષેત્રોને ફેરવવું મુશ્કેલ છે? મારા જીવનના આ ક્ષેત્રોમાં હું શરણાગતિ પર કેવી રીતે કામ કરીશ?

Self-will

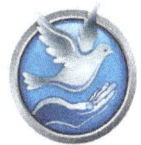

Step Three is critical because we've acted on self-will for so long, abusing our right to make choices and decisions. So what exactly is self-will? Sometimes it's total withdrawal and isolation. We end up living a very lonely and self-absorbed existence. Sometimes self-will causes us to act to the exclusion of any considerations other than what we want. We ignore the needs and feelings of others. We barrel through, stampeding over anyone who questions our right to do whatever we want. We become tornadoes, whipping through the lives of family, friends, and even strangers, totally unconscious of the path of destruction we have left behind. If circumstances aren't to our liking, we try to change them by any means necessary to achieve our aims. We try to get our way at all costs. We are so busy aggressively pursuing our impulses that we completely lose touch with our conscience and with a Higher Power. To work this step, each one of us needs to identify the ways in which we have acted on self-will.

Surrendering our self-will doesn't mean we can't pursue goals or try to make changes in our lives and the world. It doesn't mean we have to passively accept injustices to ourselves or to people for whom we're responsible. We need to differentiate between destructive self-will and constructive action.

How have I acted on self-will throughout my life? What has been the effect of my self-will on my life, and others around me?

मी आयुष्यभर स्व-इच्छेनुसार कसे वागलो? माझ्या आत्म-इच्छेचा माझ्या जीवनावर आणि माझ्या सभोवतालच्या इतरांवर काय परिणाम झाला आहे?

मैंने अपने पूरे जीवन में स्व-इच्छा पर कैसे कार्य किया है? मेरी आत्म-इच्छा का मेरे जीवन पर और मेरे आसपास के अन्य लोगों पर क्या प्रभाव पड़ा है?

મેં મારા જીવનભર સ્વ-ઇચ્છા પર કેવી રીતે કામ કર્યું છે? મારી સ્વ-ઇચ્છાની મારા જીવન પર અને મારી આસપાસના અન્ય લોકો પર શું અસર થઇ છે?

Will I have to compromise on any spiritual principles to achieve my goals? (Examples: Do I need to harm others to meet my goals, or do I have to lie or steal for my ambition)

माझे ध्येय साध्य करण्यासाठी मला कोणत्याही आध्यात्मिक तत्त्वांशी तडजोड करावी लागेल का? (उदाहरणे: माझी उद्दिष्टे पूर्ण करण्यासाठी मला इतरांना हानी पोहोचवण्याची गरज आहे का, किंवा मला माझ्या महत्त्वाकांक्षेसाठी खोटे बोलणे किंवा चोरी करणे आवश्यक आहे का)

क्या मुझे अपने लक्ष्यों को प्राप्त करने के लिए किसी आध्यात्मिक सिद्धांत से समझौता करना होगा? (उदाहरण: क्या मुझे अपने लक्ष्यों को पूरा करने के लिए दूसरों को नुकसान पहुँचाने की ज़रूरत है, या क्या मुझे अपनी महत्वाकांक्षा के लिए झूठ बोलना या चोरी करना है)

શું મારે મારા લક્ષ્યોને પ્રાપ્ત કરવા માટે કોઈ આધ્યાત્મિક સિદ્ધાંતો સાથે સમાધાન કરવું પડશે? (ઉદાહરણ: શું મારે મારા ધ્યેયો પૂરા કરવા માટે અન્ય લોકોને નુકસાન પહોંચાડવાની જરૂર છે, અથવા મારે મારી મહત્વાકાંક્ષા માટે જૂઠું બોલવું અથવા ચોરી કરવી પડશે)

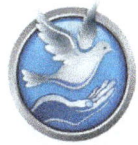

What is the difference between my will and God's will? How exactly is God's will better for me?

माझी इच्छा आणि देवाची इच्छा यात काय फरक आहे? देवाची इच्छा माझ्यासाठी नक्की कशी चांगली आहे?

मेरी इच्छा और ईश्वर की इच्छा में क्या अंतर है? परमेश्वर की इच्छा वास्तव में मेरे लिए किस प्रकार बेहतर है?

મારી ઇચ્છા અને ભગવાનની ઇચ્છા વચ્ચે શું તફાવત છે? ભગવાનની ઇચ્છા મારા માટે કેવી રીતે સારી છે?

As our understanding of a Higher Power grows and evolves, we'll find that we react differently to what goes on in our lives. We may find ourselves able to courageously face situations that used to strike fear in our hearts. We may deal with frustrations more gracefully. We may find ourselves able to pause and think about a situation before acting. We'll probably be calmer, less compulsive, and more able to see beyond the immediacy of the moment.

Turning It Over

For us to be comfortable with allowing our Higher Power to care for our lives, we will have to develop some trust. We may have no trouble turning over our addiction, but want to remain in control of the rest of our lives. We may trust our Higher Power to care for our work lives, but not our relationships. We may trust our Higher Power to care for our partners, but not our children. We may trust our Higher Power with our safety, but not our finances. Many of us have trouble letting go completely. We think we trust our Higher Power with certain

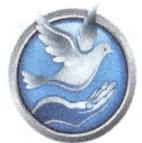

areas of our lives, but immediately take control the first time we get scared, or things aren't going the way we think they should. It's necessary for us to examine our progress in turning it over.

To turn our will and our lives over to the care of our Higher Power, we must take some kind of action. Many of us find that it works best for us to make some formal declaration on a regular basis. We may want to use the following quote from our Basic Text: "Take my will and my life. Guide me in my recovery. Show me how to live." This seems to capture the essence of Step Three for many of us. However, we can certainly feel free to find our own words, or to find a more informal way of taking action. Many of us believe that every day we abstain from using, or take suggestions from our sponsor, we are taking practical action on our decision to turn our will and lives over to the care of our Higher Power.

Spiritual Principles

We will focus first on surrender and willingness. Then we will look at how hope translates into faith and trust. Finally, we will see how the principle of commitment is tied to the Third Step.

Practicing the principle of surrender is easy for us when everything is going along as we'd like—we think. Actually, when things are going smoothly, it's more likely that we are being lulled into a belief that we're in charge, which doesn't require much "surrender." Keeping the principle of surrender to the care of the God of our understanding alive in our spirits is essential, even when things are going well.

What does it mean for me to turn my will and my life over to the care of the God of my understanding? How will allow a Higher Power to work in my life?

माझी इच्छा आणि माझे जीवन माझ्या समजूतदार देवाच्या काळजीकडे वळवण्याचा मला काय अर्थ आहे? माझ्या जीवनात उच्च शक्ती कशी कार्य करू देईल?

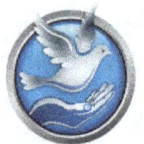

© 2024 – ANMOL JEEVAN FOUNDATION – PROPRIETARY AWARENESS & TRAINING MATERIAL FOR RECOVERING DRUG / SEX / CYBER / PORN ADDICTS, ALCOHOLICS, GAMBLERS, PSYCHIATRIC ILLNESS AND PERSONALITY DISORDERS.

मेरे लिए अपनी इच्छा और अपने जीवन को अपनी समझ के परमेश्वर की देखभाल में सौंपने का क्या अर्थ है? कैसे एक उच्च शक्ति को मेरे जीवन में काम करने देगा?

મારી ઇચ્છા અને મારા જીવનને મારી સમજણના ભગવાનની સંભાળમાં ફેરવવાનો મારા માટે શું અર્થ છે? મારા જીવનમાં ઉચ્ચ શક્તિ કેવી રીતે કામ કરવા દેશે?

_____
_____
_____
_____
_____
_____
_____
_____
_____
_____
_____
_____
_____
_____
_____
_____
_____
_____
_____
_____
_____
_____
_____
_____
_____

How have I become "Willing" in my recovery now? How have "Hope", "Faith", and "Trust" become positive forces in my life?

मी आता माझ्या पुनर्प्राप्तीमध्ये "इच्छुक" कसे झालो? माझ्या आयुष्यात "आशा", "विश्वास" आणि "श्रद्धा" या सकारात्मक शक्ती कशा बनल्या आहेत?

अब मैं अपने सुधार में "इच्छुक" कैसे बन गया हूँ? कैसे "आशा", "विश्वास" और " श्रद्धा" मेरे जीवन में सकारात्मक शक्ति बन गए हैं?

હવે મારી પુનઃપ્રાપ્તિમાં હું કેવી રીતે "ઇચ્છુક" બન્યો? મારા જીવનમાં "આશા", "વિશ્વાસ" અને " વખાણ" કેવી રીતે સકારાત્મક શક્તિઓ બની છે?

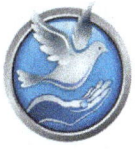
© 2024 – ANMOL JEEVAN FOUNDATION – PROPRIETARY AWARENESS & TRAINING MATERIAL FOR RECOVERING DRUG / SEX / CYBER / PORN ADDICTS, ALCOHOLICS, GAMBLERS, PSYCHIATRIC ILLNESS AND PERSONALITY DISORDERS.

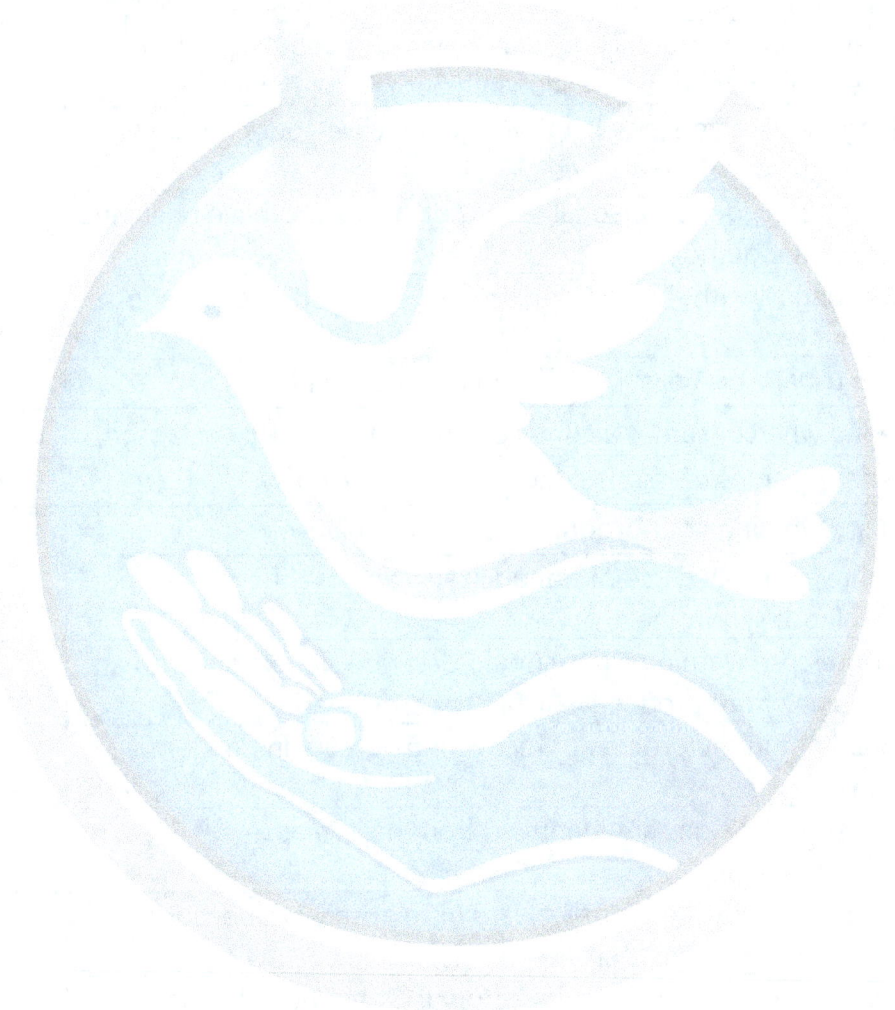

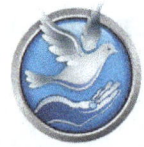

© 2024 – ANMOL JEEVAN FOUNDATION – PROPRIETARY AWARENESS & TRAINING MATERIAL FOR RECOVERING DRUG / SEX / CYBER / PORN ADDICTS, ALCOHOLICS, GAMBLERS, PSYCHIATRIC ILLNESS AND PERSONALITY DISORDERS.

STEP THREE TEST

Sr.	Questions	True	False
1	It is not the event but your reaction to the event that can make you dysfunctional because of post acute withdrawal.		
2	The best way to manage stress is to solve the problems causing it.		
3	Spiritual discipline is doing specific things on a regular basis to increase your conscious contact with your Higher Power.		
4	Working the Twelve Steps helps you to increase your conscious contact with your Higher Power.		
5	Journaling provides a personal record of where you have been and where you are going.		
6	Relapse begins with the first drink/drug s are used after a period of abstinence.		
7	Relapse usually occurs suddenly and unexpectedly.		
8	Someone who consumes alcohol, even accidentally, has relapsed.		
9	The warning signs of relapse develop subconsciously.		
10	If you are working your program, you won't relapse.		
11	Moderate, controlled use of tranquilizers can ease the progression of the relapse syndrome.		
12	A list of relapse warning signs should describe signals that you are moving away from productive living towards relapse.		
13	If you are not in the process of recovering you are in danger of relapsing.		
14	Relapse warning signs are identified from past relapse experiences.		
15	You must become consciously aware of relapse warning signs before you can change them.		
16	The main purpose for regular inventory is to help you become better educated about stages of recovery.		
17	Part of relapse prevention planning is educating the people you are close to about addiction and your relapse warning signs.		

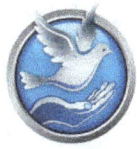

© 2024 – ANMOL JEEVAN FOUNDATION – PROPRIETARY AWARENESS & TRAINING MATERIAL FOR RECOVERING DRUG / SEX / CYBER / PORN ADDICTS, ALCOHOLICS, GAMBLERS, PSYCHIATRIC ILLNESS AND PERSONALITY DISORDERS.

18	You will need to change your relapse prevention plan from time to time.		
19	Relapse means starting over in recovery.		
20	The main purpose of a good recovery program is to help you identify relapse warning signs.		

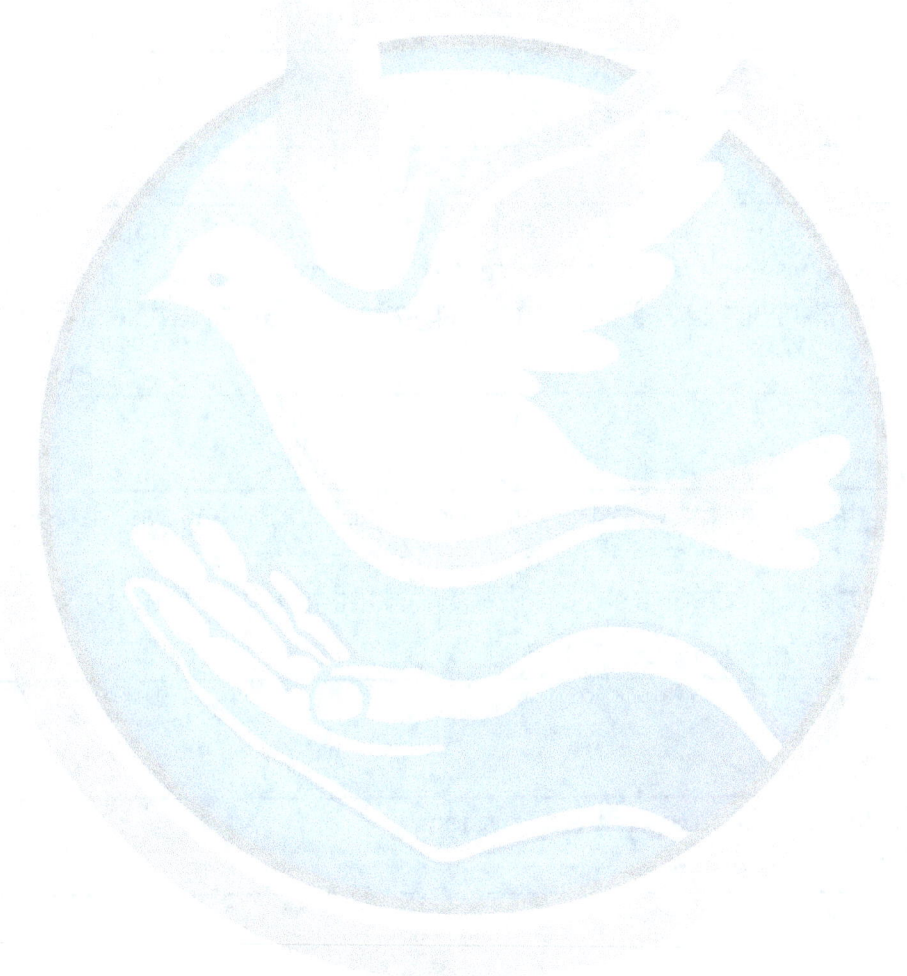

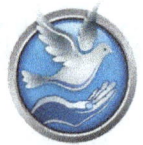

© 2024 – ANMOL JEEVAN FOUNDATION – PROPRIETARY AWARENESS & TRAINING MATERIAL FOR RECOVERING DRUG / SEX / CYBER / PORN ADDICTS, ALCOHOLICS, GAMBLERS, PSYCHIATRIC ILLNESS AND PERSONALITY DISORDERS.

FINANCIAL MISMANAGEMENT INVENTORY

- Which year did you start your addiction (First time of consuming alcohol, substance or gambling). What was your age at that time.

आपने किस वर्ष अपना व्यसन शुरू किया (शराब या ड्रग्स के सेवन का पहली बार। जुए का पहला समय, वेश्याओं के साथ सेक्स)। उस समय आपकी उम्र क्या थी?

- Total addiction duration –

आप कितने साल से नशे की लत में हैं

- How many times have you been hospitalized due to your addiction. How many times have you visited a rehabilitation centre for detox.

आपकी लत के कारण आप कितनी बार अस्पताल में भर्ती हुए हैं। कितनी बार आपने डिटॉक्स के पुनर्वास केंद्र का दौरा किया है।

- What was the approximate cost of every hospitalization. What was the cost of medicines and the medical tests. What was the total expense -

हर अस्पताल में भर्ती का खर्च क्या था। दवाओं और चिकित्सा परीक्षणों का खर्च क्या था। इन अस्पतालों और दवाओं का कुल खर्च क्या था

- Cost of total rehabilitation centre admissions –

कुल पुनर्वास केंद्र प्रवेश की खर्च -

- What is the approximate cost of alcohol and addictive substances consumed till date –

आज तक सेवन किए गए अल्कोहल और नशीले पदार्थों की अनुमानित खर्च क्या है -

[ ]

- What financial opportunities did you lose because of your addiction, gambling or alcoholism. (Job, Business, Investment, Training etc.). Describe in detail.
आपकी लत, जुआ या शराब की वजह से आपको किन वित्तीय अवसरों से हाथ धोना पड़ा। (नौकरी, व्यवसाय, निवेश, प्रशिक्षण आदि)

[ ]

- Number of years of unemployment –
बेरोजगारी के वर्षों की संख्या -

[ ]

- During Addiction what amount of loans have you incurred. What amount of these loans taken, have been cleared / repaid by your family –
व्यसन के दौरान किस राशि के लिए कितना ऋण लिया गया है। आपके द्वारा लिए गए इन ऋणों की कितनी राशि, आपके परिवार द्वारा चुका दी गई है -

[ ]

- What is the amount of unpaid loans now -
आपकी लत के कारण अब अवैतनिक ऋण की राशि क्या है

[ ]

- How much money did you make by cheating, fooliong or defrauding other innocents during your addiction -
अपनी लत के दौरान आपने दूसरों को धोखा देकर कितना पैसा कमाया।

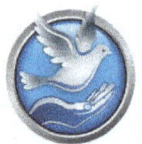 © 2024 – ANMOL JEEVAN FOUNDATION – PROPRIETARY AWARENESS & TRAINING MATERIAL FOR RECOVERING DRUG / SEX / CYBER / PORN ADDICTS, ALCOHOLICS, GAMBLERS, PSYCHIATRIC ILLNESS AND PERSONALITY DISORDERS.

- Family assets / property / business lost due to cost of addiction – Gold ornaments of wife / daughters, FD / Savings / Pension / PF liquidated, Shop / house / plot / shares -

आपके पीने या ड्रग्स के कारण पारिवारिक संपत्ति क्या खो गई। (पत्नी / बेटियां सोने के गहने, घर, दुकान, जमीन, शेयर, जमा पैसा, पेंशन)

- Cost of relationship losses (Divorce, Legal fees, Police matters) -
आपके खराब संबंधों के मुद्दों के कारण खर्च क्या था। (तलाक, कानूनी शुल्क, पुलिस मामला)

- Cost of Jail-Bail, Bribes, Setting –
जेल-बेल (जेल-जमानत), राजनीतिक, रिश्वत, रिश्वत, सेटिंग के खर्च -

- Money wasted due to grandiosity in addiction – Giving gifts to please people, Paying for friends, Dance bar / Prostitution / Girl friends, Gambling

तूमतड़ाक (भव्य) खर्चों पर पैसा बर्बाद - दोस्तों शराब और ड्रग्स के लिए भुगतान करना -- डांस बार, वेश्याओं पर खर्च, जुआ, लड़कियों को इंप्रेस करना, दूसरों को प्रभावित करने के लिए महंगे उपहार खरीदना।

- Total cost of your addiction, bad habits, wasted expenses over the years. Describe and other expenses incurred also.

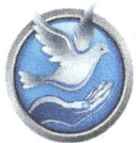

© 2024 – ANMOL JEEVAN FOUNDATION – PROPRIETARY AWARENESS & TRAINING MATERIAL FOR RECOVERING DRUG / SEX / CYBER / PORN ADDICTS, ALCOHOLICS, GAMBLERS, PSYCHIATRIC ILLNESS AND PERSONALITY DISORDERS.

इन वर्षों में आपकी लत, शराब और बुरी आदतों पर कुल कितना रुपया बर्बाद हुआ है. वर्णन करें और नशे की वजह से आपके द्वारा किए गए अन्य खर्चों को भी जोड़ें।वर्णन करें और नशे की वजह से आपके द्वारा किए गए अन्य खर्चों को भी जोड़ें।

[ ]

- Future expenses as result of your addiction

भविष्य का खर्च

- At the moment what physical & mentals ailments / conditions / complaints do you have -

अब आप किस बीमारी से पीड़ित हैं? - शारीरिक और मानसिक।

[ ]

- What amount is required for treating your current medical problems - Surgery, Medical Tests, Doctor fees, Medicines etc.

इन चिकित्सा बीमारियों के इलाज के लिए अनुमानित खर्च क्या है। (मेडिकल टेस्ट। सर्जरी। दवाएं। डॉक्टर की फीस।)

[ ]

- How much more money do you think is required to complete your rehabilitation & for you to stand on your own feet.

आपको अपने पैरों पर खड़े होने के लिए और अधिक खर्चों की आवश्यकता होती है। आपको क्या लगता है कि इसके लिए कुल कितनी राशि की आवश्यकता है।

[ ]

This is a material balance sheet of what you have wasted / lost in life. Describe how you feel after writing & reviewing this. What are your realizations.

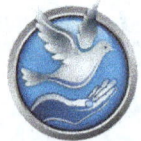 © 2024 – ANMOL JEEVAN FOUNDATION – PROPRIETARY AWARENESS & TRAINING MATERIAL FOR RECOVERING DRUG / SEX / CYBER / PORN ADDICTS, ALCOHOLICS, GAMBLERS, PSYCHIATRIC ILLNESS AND PERSONALITY DISORDERS.

यह आपकी लत का लेखा-जोखा है। आपके अहसास क्या हैं?

इस खाते को लिखने और उसकी समीक्षा करने के बाद आप कैसा महसूस करते हैं। कृपया अपनी संबंधित टिप्पणियाँ या नीचे महसूस करें।

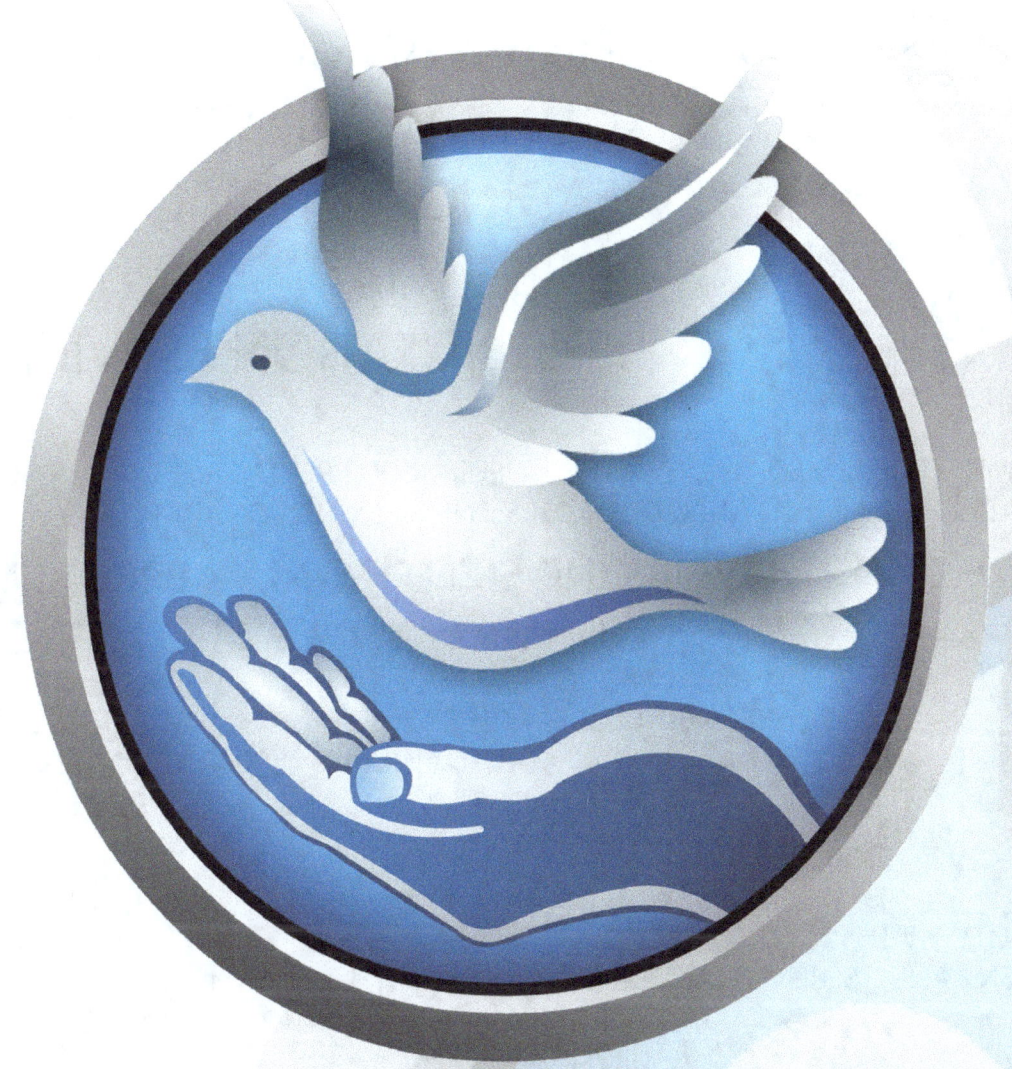

ANMOL JEEVAN FOUNDATION

CENTRE FOR DE-ADDICTION, MENTAL ILLNESS TREATMENT & PSYCHIATRIC CARE

PSYCHIATRIC HOSPITAL PERMANENT REGN. NO. 5/2023 & 17/2023

FRIENDS OF THE FALLEN AND GUIDES TO THOSE ON THE PATH OF RECOVERY

WE ARE SPECIALISTS IN DEALING WITH ALCOHOLISM, DRUG ABUSE, SEX / CYBER / PORN ADDICTION, AND GAMBLING. WE ENCOURAGE YOU TO SEEK PROFESSIONAL HELP BEFORE IT IS TOO LATE.

WWW.ANMOLJEEVAN.ORG / ANMOLJEEVANWELLNESS@GMAIL.COM

+91 9158071666 / 9666 & +91 8080 8989 41/42

THE ANMOL JEEVAN FOUNDATION IS INDIA'S LEADING PROVIDER OF RESIDENTIAL REHABILITATION SERVICES.

OUR LICENSED MEDICAL FACILITIES OFFER COMPREHENSIVE CARE FOR THE TREATMENT OF PSYCHIATRIC DISORDERS AND ALL KINDS OF ADDICTIONS.

WE DON'T HAVE A ONE-SIZE-FITS-ALL APPROACH.

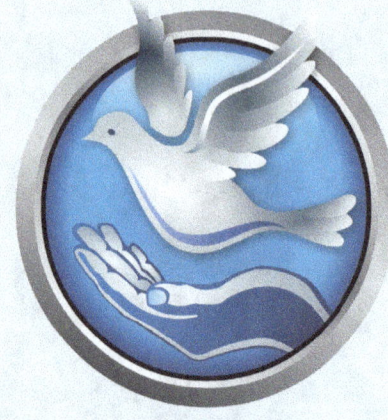

WE UNDERSTAND & RESPECT THAT EVERY CLIENT IS UNIQUE. OUR TEAM OF DEDICATED PROFESSIONALS INCLUDE —BEST IN CLASS PSYCHIATRISTS, CLINICAL AND BEHAVIOURAL PSYCHOTHERAPISTS, COUNSELLORS, PHYSICIANS AND DE-ADDICTION SPECIALISTS.

WE OFFER •COMPLETELY AIR CONDITIONED FACILITY, WITH 24X7X365 RESIDENT MEDICAL OFFICERS & PHARMACISTS •A GREEN AND SERENE LANDSCAPED ENVIRONMENT •AMBULANCE SERVICE •ISOLATED DETOXIFICATION CENTRE •CCTV SURVEILLANCE & PHYSICAL SECURITY •LAUNDRY FACILITY •HOT-COLD RO-FILTERED WATER IN EACH ROOM •INDOOR (TT, BOARD GAMES, CARROM, & POOL) & OUTDOOR GAMES (VOLLEYBALL, CRICKET & SOCCER) •FULLY EQUIPPED GYMNASIUM •WHOLESOME VARIETY OF CONTINENTAL AND INDIAN CUISINES (BASED ON NUTRITIONIST RECOMMENDATIONS AND SPECIAL NEEDS) •INDIVIDUAL AND GROUP THERAPY •TECHNOLOGY EQUIPPED LECTURE HALL WITH A FULLY WI-FI CAMPUS

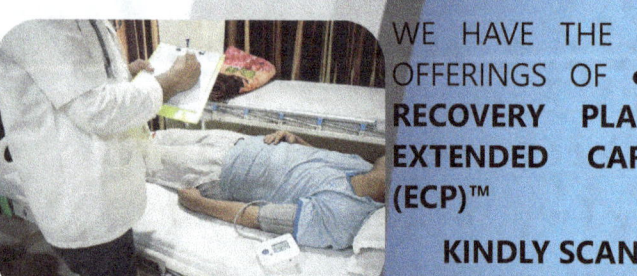

WE HAVE THE MOST UNIQUE OFFERINGS OF •**ACCELARATED RECOVERY PLAN (ARP)**™ •**EXTENDED CARE PROGRAM (ECP)**™

KINDLY SCAN THE BARCODE FOR DIRECTIONS. SCHEDULE A VISIT WITH US FOR A WALKTHROUGH

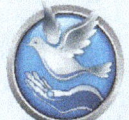 ANMOL JEEVAN FOUNDATION – PSYCHIATRIC HOSPITAL & NURSING HOME SPECIALIZED IN DE-ADDICTION THERAPY, MENTAL ILLNESS AND PSYCHIATRIC CARE – PERMANENT REGISTRATION NO. 5/2023

FOR THOSE FAMILIES … WHO HAVE AN ALCOHOLIC, ADDICT, GAMBLER, ANY PERSON SUFFERING FROM MENTAL OR PSYCHIATRIC ILLNESS, OR PERSONALITY DISORDERS IN THEIR LIVES
<u>45 DAY – ACCELERATED RECOVERY PROGRAM</u>

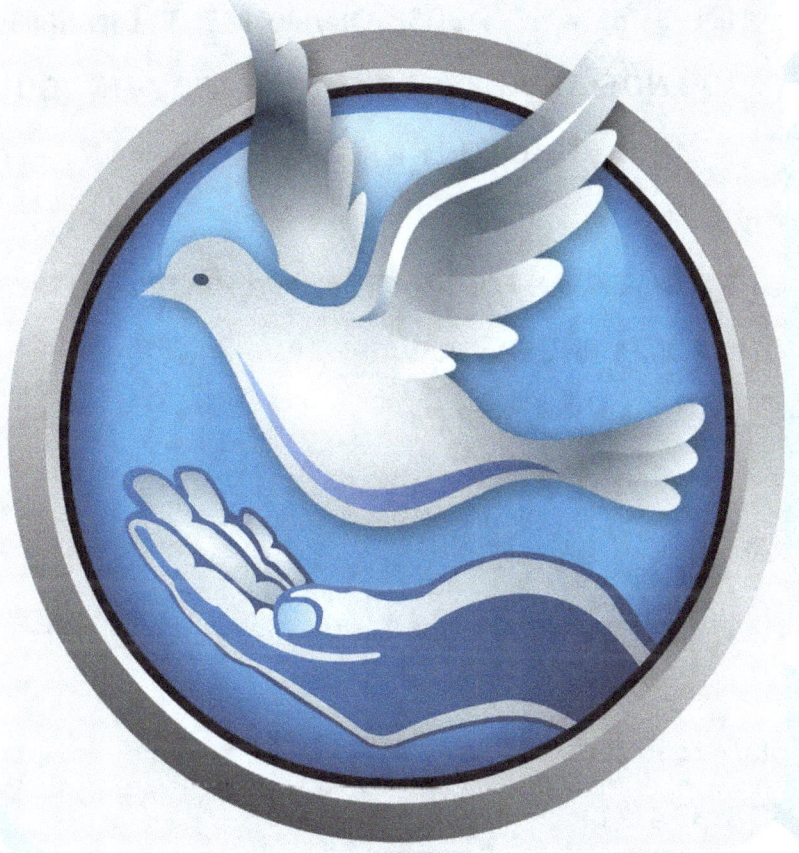

DO YOU HAVE SOMEONE (THAT YOU LOVE) IN YOUR LIFE WHO IS CONSUMING ALCOHOL OR DRUGS – THAT SEEMS TO BE OUT OF HIS CONTROL?

DID YOU KNOW THAT ANY OF <u>ALCOHOL OR DRUG ADDICTION IS A DISEASE</u>? – AND THAT THIS IS A LIFE-LONG CHRONIC CONDITION, WHICH LEADS TO LONG-TERM SOCIO-PSYCHO-ECONOMIC EFFECTS?

<u>THIS IS A SELF-HELP GUIDE FOR THOSE FAMILIES SEEKING TO HELP A "VERY SICK PERSON", AND OVERCOME ANY OF THESE MALADIES</u>

© 2023 - A WELLBEING GUIDE FOR THE FAMILIES & FRIENDS OF ALCOHOL, DRUG, SEX ADDICTS, AND COMPULSIVE GAMBLERS BY THE ANMOL JEEVAN FOUNDATION™
ANMOLJEEVANWELNESS@GMAIL.COM WWW.ANMOLWELNESS.ORG
+91 915807 1666 / 915807 9666 & +91 8080 8989 41/42

 ANMOL JEEVAN FOUNDATION – PSYCHIATRIC HOSPITAL & NURSING HOME SPECIALIZED IN DE-ADDICTION THERAPY, MENTAL ILLNESS AND PSYCHIATRIC CARE – PERMANENT REGISTRATION NO. 5/2023

SEEK HELP, BEFORE ITS TOO LATE – WE ARE HERE FOR YOU.

ALCOHOL, DRUGS, GAMBLING, SEX OR ANY OTHER SUBSTANCE AND NON-SUBSTANCE ABUSE, OR ANY MENTAL ILLNESS …

DO NOT STRUGGLE ALONE! – WE ARE WITH YOU!

REACH OUT TO US 24 X 7 X 365

ANMOL JEEVAN FOUNDATION PSYCHIATRIC HOSPITAL

RAJDOOT WADI, PURNUKPADA, VAJRESHWARI ROAD,

SHIRAVLI, POST PAROL, VIRAR (EAST),

TALUKA – VASAI, DISTRICT – PALGHAR – 401 303.

MAHARASHTRA, INDIA.

ANMOLJEEVANWELNESS@GMAIL.COM

WWW.ANMOLWELNESS.ORG

+91 915807 1666 / 915807 9666 &

+91 8080 8989 41/42

ALSO FIND AND CONNECT WITH US ON SOCIAL MEDIA – FACEBOOK AND INSTAGRAM

 ANMOL JEEVAN FOUNDATION – PSYCHIATRIC HOSPITAL & NURSING HOME SPECIALIZED IN DE-ADDICTION THERAPY, MENTAL ILLNESS AND PSYCHIATRIC CARE – PERMANENT REGISTRATION NO. 5/2023

WHAT IS THE ANMOL JEEVAN ACCELERATED RECOVERY PROGRAM?

ANMOL JEEVAN FOUNDATION OFFERS AN UNIQUE 45 DAY RECOVERY PLAN THAT IS BASED ON BEST PRACTICES OF THE DIAGNOSTIC AND STATISTICAL MANUAL OF MENTAL DISORDERS (DSM-IV), THE GORSKI-CENAPS© MODEL OF RECOVERY AND RELAPSE PREVENTION, CENTRE FOR SUBSTANCE ABUSE TREATMENT (CSAT, USA), THE HAZELDEN DEVELOPMENTAL MODEL OF RECOVERY (DMR), THE 12 STEPS OF ALCOHOLICS / NARCOTICS ANONYMOUS (AA / NA), AND THE EXPERIENCE OF THOUSANDS OF RECOVERING ADDICTS AROUND THE WORLD.

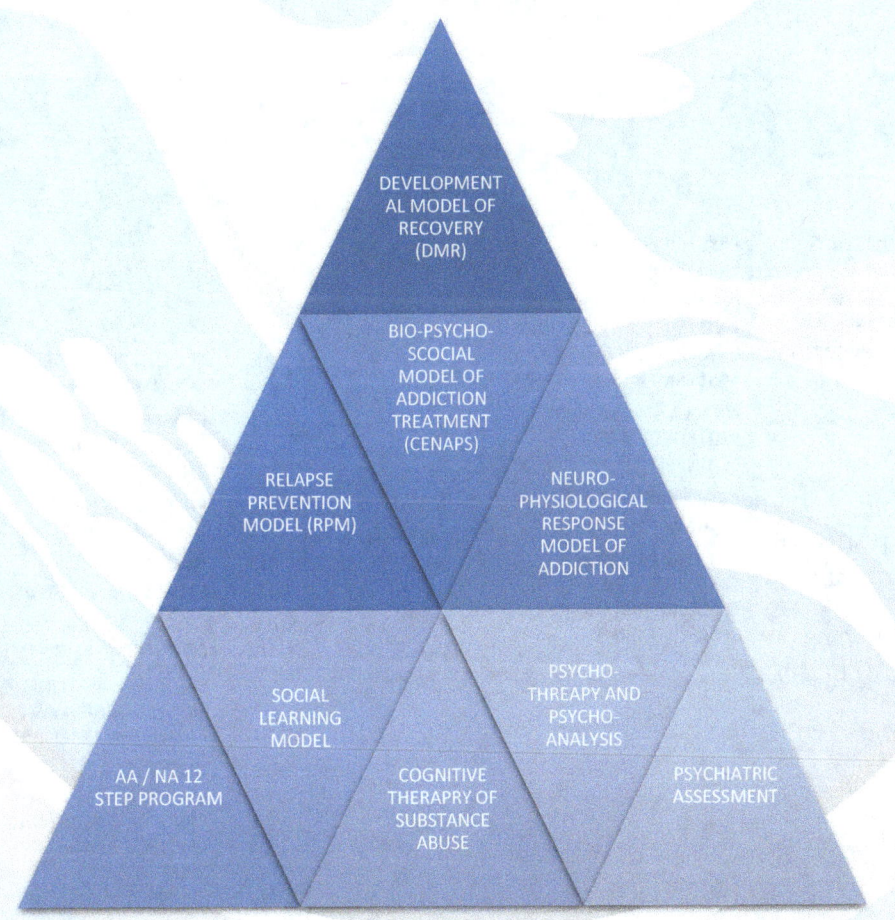

© 2023 - A WELLBEING GUIDE FOR THE FAMILIES & FRIENDS OF ALCOHOL, DRUG, SEX ADDICTS, AND COMPULSIVE GAMBLERS BY THE ANMOL JEEVAN FOUNDATION™
ANMOLJEEVANWELNESS@GMAIL.COM WWW.ANMOLWELNESS.ORG
+91 915807 1666 / 915807 9666 & +91 8080 8989 41/42

 ANMOL JEEVAN FOUNDATION – PSYCHIATRIC HOSPITAL & NURSING HOME SPECIALIZED IN DE-ADDICTION THERAPY, MENTAL ILLNESS AND PSYCHIATRIC CARE – PERMANENT REGISTRATION NO. 5/2023

WE ADOPT A **3 DIMENSIONAL APPROACH** TO TREATMENT OF THE ADDICT PATIENTS –

- PRE-TREATMENT DETOXIFICATION
- PHYSICAL & MENTAL ASSESSMENT
- CONTINUOUS COUNSELLING, PSYCHOLOGICAL ASSESSMENT & 12 STEP PROGRAM

THE 45 DAYS ARE STRATEGICALLY BROKEN DOWN INTO 4 PHASES –

WEEKS 1 & 2

- PATIENT BACKGROUND AND HISTORY
- FAMILY COUNSELLING - ADDICTION DISEASE CONCEPT, TREATMENT PATTERN AND CONCERNS
- PATIENT DETOXIFICATION
- PHYSIOLOGICAL MEDICAL ASSESSMENT
- ECG
- PATHOLOGICAL INVESTIGATIONS
- PSYCHIATRIC EVALUATION
- PHARMACOLOGICAL REGIME
- DIET DETERMINATION
- PHYSICAL WORKOUT AND GROUP THERAPY
- FAMILY FEEDBACK - BIO-PSYCHO-SOCIAL BY PSYCHIATRIST AND COUNSELLOR

WEEKS 3 & 4

- PSYCHIATRIC RE-EVALUATION
- INDIVIDUAL COUNSELLING AND THERAPY BASED ON PSYCHOLOGICAL ASSESSMENTS
- AA / NA STEP WORKING WITH DEDICATED COUNSELLOR
- ASSIGNMENTS BASED ON IQ AND APTITUDE
- PATIENT PROGRESS TRACKING & FAMILY FEEDBACK VIA VIDEO CONFERENCING

WEEK 4 & 5

- ALIGNMENT OF PATIENT TO THE 12 STEP PROGRAM
- PARTICIPATION IN THE IN-HOUSE AA/NA MEETINGS
- PERSONAL COUNSELLING BASED ON PSYCHOLOGICAL EVALUATION
- FAMILY VISIT & FACTUAL CONFRONTATION (FCC)
- ADVANCED STEP WORKING, AND SPIRITUAL DEVELOPMENT

WEEK 6 - DISCHARGE

- FCC OUTPUT BASED COUNSELLING
- REASSESSMENT OF PATIENT READINESS AND WILLINGNESS
- PREPARING FOR THE OUTSIDE WORLD - ACCEPT NEW REALITIES
- RELAPSE MANAGEMENT PROGRAM
- COUNSELLOR SIGN OFF
- JOINT COUNSELLING SESSION - FAMILY & PATIENT RE-INTEGRATION
- GUIDANCE ON MAINTENANCE PHASE - AA / NA + AL-ANON / NAR-ANON OR ALA-TEEN MEETINGS

© 2023 - A WELLBEING GUIDE FOR THE FAMILIES & FRIENDS OF ALCOHOL, DRUG, SEX ADDICTS, AND COMPULSIVE GAMBLERS BY THE ANMOL JEEVAN FOUNDATION™
ANMOLJEEVANWELNESS@GMAIL.COM WWW.ANMOLWELNESS.ORG
+91 915807 1666 / 915807 9666 & +91 8080 8989 41/42

 ANMOL JEEVAN FOUNDATION – PSYCHIATRIC HOSPITAL & NURSING HOME SPECIALIZED IN DE-ADDICTION THERAPY, MENTAL ILLNESS AND PSYCHIATRIC CARE – PERMANENT REGISTRATION NO. 5/2023

PHYSIOLOGICAL EVALUATIONS	PHYSIATRIC EVALUATION	PSYCHOLOGICAL EVALATIONS	PERSONAL COUNSELLING

• COVID TESTING
• DRUG / ALCOHOL TESTING
• MEDICAL ASSESSMENT
• ECG
• FULL BLOOD & URINE PANEL
  • LIVER, KIDNEY FUNCTION TESTS
  • THYROID TESTS
  • BLOOD COUNT ANALYSIS
  • SUGAR CONTROL ANALYSIS
	• MENTAL AND EMOTIONAL STATE
	• PAIN MANAGMENT
	• (SUBSTANCE) CRAVING CONTROL
	• MOOD ANALYSIS
	• PHARMA SUBSTITUTION / REPLACEMENT
		• MMPI/ MCMI
		• HTP
		• TAT
		• RORSHARC / INK BLOT
		• K10 - DASS 21 - DEPRESSION / ANXIETY ANALYSIS
		• DAST
		• AUDIT
		• PERSONALITY ANALYSIS
		• AWARE RELAPSE ANALSYS
			• PATIENT ALIGNMENT STATUS & GENERAL WELL-BEING
			• PATIENT AUTOBIOGRAPHY - LIFE HIGHLIGHT ANALYSIS
			• ANGER - FEAR - GUILT ANALYSIS
			• AA / NA 12 STEP WORKING
			• DAILY THOUGHT- EMOTION & CHARACTER DEFECT INVENTORY

THE **POST-DISCHARGE FOLLOW UP** COMPROMISES OF –

- 1 CLIENT VISIT + 48 HOUR STAY AT THE CENTRE – TO REVISIT THE 12 STEP RECOVERY PROGRAM WITH THE COUNSELLOR, AS WELL AS A REVISION OF THE RELAPSE PREVENTION PROGRAM (RPP). THIS IS DONE 15 DAYS POST DISCHARGE.
- 2 CLIENT + FAMILY VISITS TO THE CENTRE – FOR A PSYCHIATRIC FOLLOW UP, AND TO SEEK ADVISE FROM THE COUNSELLORS ON MAINTAINING RECOVERY. THESE VISITS ARE TO BE SCHEDULED BETWEEN 30-60 DAYS POST DISCHARGE, BY TAKING A PRIOR APPOINTMENT FROM THE ADMINISTRATION DEPARTMENT.

© 2023 - A WELLBEING GUIDE FOR THE FAMILIES & FRIENDS OF ALCOHOL, DRUG, SEX ADDICTS, AND COMPULSIVE GAMBLERS BY THE ANMOL JEEVAN FOUNDATION™
ANMOLJEEVANWELNESS@GMAIL.COM WWW.ANMOLWELNESS.ORG
+91 915807 1666 / 915807 9666 & +91 8080 8989 41/42

 ANMOL JEEVAN FOUNDATION – PSYCHIATRIC HOSPITAL & NURSING HOME SPECIALIZED IN DE-ADDICTION THERAPY, MENTAL ILLNESS AND PSYCHIATRIC CARE – PERMANENT REGISTRATION NO. 5/2023

WHAT DOES ANMOL JEEVAN PROMISE TO OFFER?

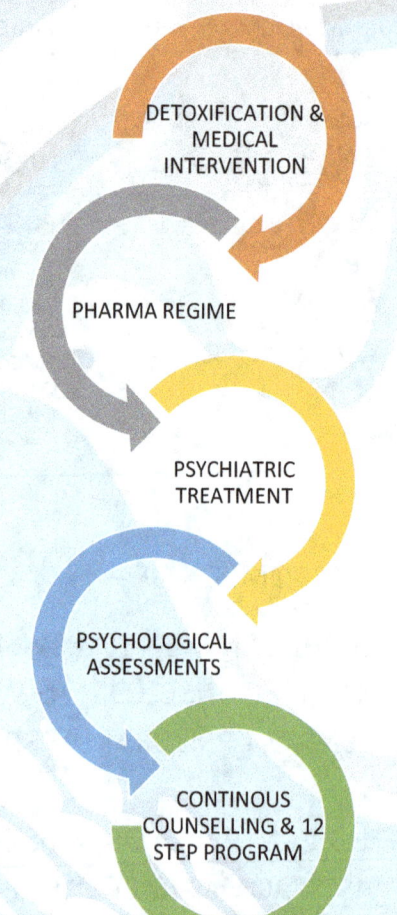

AT ANMOL JEEVAN WE FIRMLY BELIEVE THAT –

- NO TWO ADDICTS ARE THE SAME, THERE IS NO ONE-SIZE-FITS-ALL TREATMENT
- EVERY ADDICT COMES TO US WITH A UNIQUE PAST, MENTAL RESERVATIONS AND EMOTIONAL STATE OF MIND
- EVERY ADDICT DESERVES RESPECT AND A HELPING HAND – HE IS NOT TO BE DRAGGED THROUGH THE MUD, OR SHAMED FOR THIS PAST
- HOPE-FILLED ADDICTS AND STRONG FAMILIES ARE MOST LIKELY TO INTEGRATE AND PROSPER
- THE REHAB SHOULD BE JUST LIKE A "HOME, AWAY FROM HOME"

WE START OUR ADMISSION PROCEDURE WITH THE PROCESS OF "**DETOXIFICATION**" AND THOROUGH **PHYSIOLOGICAL AND PATHOLOGICAL INVESTIGATIONS** – THUS DETERMINING THE FITNESS OF THE PATIENT TO START THE PROGRAM. WE ALLOW AS MUCH TIME AS THE PATIENT NEEDS TO STAND HIS GROUND FIRMLY, AND BE ACCUSTOMED TO THE NEW CONDITIONS OF THE REHAB.

<u>THE PHARMACOLOGICAL (MEDICINES) REGIME IS FINALIZED AFTER A DETAILED PSYCHIATRIC ASSESSMENT.</u> WE ASCERTAIN MENTAL AILMENTS AND DISORDERS, OR ANY OTHER "SPECIAL NEEDS" OF THE PATIENT. <u>THE DIET AND PHYSICAL ACTIVITY PLAN OF THE PATIENT IS ALSO FINALIZED BY THE MEDICAL TEAMS.</u>

WE OFFER WHOLESOME MEALS THAT ARE DESIGNED TO FULFIL THE NUTRITION AND NOURISHMENT NEEDS EVERY PATIENT. "SPECIAL NEEDS" PATIENTS, DIABETICS OR THOSE SUFFERING FROM LIVER AND DIGESTIVE AILMENTS ARE PROVIDED WITH MEALS TO SUIT THEIR NEEDS AND INTAKE IS MONITORED BY THE ONSITE MEDICAL TEAM. SUMMARY OF OUR MEAL PROGRAM WOULD BE –

© 2023 - A WELLBEING GUIDE FOR THE FAMILIES & FRIENDS OF ALCOHOL, DRUG, SEX ADDICTS, AND COMPULSIVE GAMBLERS BY THE ANMOL JEEVAN FOUNDATION™
ANMOLJEEVANWELNESS@GMAIL.COM WWW.ANMOLWELNESS.ORG
+91 915807 1666 / 915807 9666 & +91 8080 8989 41/42

ANMOL JEEVAN FOUNDATION – PSYCHIATRIC HOSPITAL & NURSING HOME SPECIALIZED IN DE-ADDICTION THERAPY, MENTAL ILLNESS AND PSYCHIATRIC CARE – PERMANENT REGISTRATION NO. 5/2023

- VARIETY OF VEGETARIAN & NON-VEGETARIAN MEALS
- EGGS – BOILED OR FRIED TWICE A WEEK
- SPECIALITY FOOD – CHINESE, CONTINENTAL AND INDIAN OCCASIONALLY
- JAIN MEALS
- MILK (WITH BOURNVITA / HORLICKS) – TWICE A DAY
- DIGESTIVE BISCUITS / PACKAGED SNACKS FOR IN-ROOM CONSUMPTION
- DAILY EVENING REFRESHMENTS WITH TEA OR COFFEE
- SEASONAL FRUITS / FRUIT JUICES / SOFT DRINKS
- CAKES AND DESERTS ON SPECIAL OCCASIONS AND FESTIVALS

ALL MEALS ARE FRESHLY COOKED AND SERVED.

RECREATION AND GROOMING ACTIVITIES INCLUDE –

- OUTDOOR SPORTS SUCH AS VOLLEYBALL, CRICKET, BADMINTON
- INDOOR SPORTS SUCH AS CAROM, CHESS, BILLIARDS / POOL
- HAIR SALON AND SPA – HAIR CUTTING / DYING / STYLING, SHAVING, AND MASSAGE
- LIBRARY – RICH IN AA / NA LITERATURE, FICTION AND NON-FICTION BOOKS, SELF HELP GUIDES, NOVELS, INSPIRATIONAL AND MOTIVATIONAL TEXTS
- MUSICAL INSTRUMENTS
- PERIODIC FUN ACTIVITIES LIKE HOUSIE, MUSICAL CHAIRS, DANCE
- YOGA, PT EXERCISES, STRETCHING, CHAIR / SITTING EXERCISES, MEDITATION AND ZUMBA – EITHER IS DONE ON A DAILY BASIS

THE ROOM AND INFRASTRUCTURE FACILITIES INCLUDE –

- SPACIOUS AND AIR-CONDITIONED ROOMS
- ATTACHED WASHROOM PER ROOM EQUIPPED WITH GEYSER AND SHOWER
- DAILY LAUNDRY PICK UP / DROP SERVICE
- BASIC TOILETRIES ARE PROVIDED IN-CENTRE
- DAILY ROOM SANITATION AND MOSQUITO FOGGING
- HOT-COLD DRINKING WATER DISPENSER
- TV WITH TATA SKY DTH
- READING AND STUDY TABLE
- 24X7 CCTV SURVEILLANCE, SECURITY TEAMS WITH WALKY-TALKIES
- ONE STAFF MEMBER PER ROOM
- RESIDENT MEDICAL OFFICER AND PHARMACIST

WE HAVE A TEAM OF EXPERT PROFESSIONALS TO ENSURE OVERALL RECOVERY AND MONITOR THE PROGRESS OF EVERY PATIENT –

- THE DETOXIFICATION CENTRE IS EQUIPPED WITH ECG MACHINES AND RESPIRATORY EQUIPMENT

© 2023 - A WELLBEING GUIDE FOR THE FAMILIES & FRIENDS OF ALCOHOL, DRUG, SEX ADDICTS, AND COMPULSIVE GAMBLERS BY THE ANMOL JEEVAN FOUNDATION™
ANMOLJEEVANWELNESS@GMAIL.COM WWW.ANMOLWELNESS.ORG
+91 915807 1666 / 915807 9666 & +91 8080 8989 41/42

 **ANMOL JEEVAN FOUNDATION – PSYCHIATRIC HOSPITAL & NURSING HOME SPECIALIZED IN DE-ADDICTION THERAPY, MENTAL ILLNESS AND PSYCHIATRIC CARE – PERMANENT REGISTRATION NO. 5/2023**

- IN-CENTRE PHARMACY FOR ADMINISTERING MEDICINES, INJECTABLE DRUGS AND 24X7 EMERGENCY RESPONSE IN CASE OF PATIENT DISTRESS
- DEDICATED AMBULANCE FOR EMERGENCY PATIENT TRANSPORT – AVAILABLE 24X7 ON PREMISE
- BEST IN CLASS PSYCHIATRIC DOCTORS ATTACHED
- TEAM OF PSYCHOLOGISTS TO A WIDE PANEL OF PSYCHOLOGICAL ASSESSMENTS
- DEDICATED COUNSELLORS ASSIGNED TO EACH PATIENT, WHO GUIDE THEM THROUGH THE 12 STEP PROGRAM AND ASSIST THEM IN EVERY STEP OF DE-ADDICT AND RELAPSE PREVENTION

STRATEGIC ALLIANCES WITH HOSPITALS, PATHOLOGY LABORATORIES AND MENTAL TREATMENT FACILITIES FOR –

- X-RAYS
- BLOOD / URINE / COVID TESTS
- ECT – ELECTRO OR CHEMICAL IMBALANCE TREATMENTS
- DENTAL TREATMENT
- OPHTHALMOLOGIST (EYE DOCTOR) AND DERMATOLOGIST (SKIN DOCTOR)
- BONE-MUSCLE TREATMENTS, FRACTURE PLASTERING ETC …

THE DAILY ROUTINE OF PATIENTS STRICTLY MONITORED BY THE IN-HOUSE STAFF. STARTING FROM BASIC HYGIENE CHECKS TO TRACKING PROGRESS IN THE 12 STEP PROGRAM IS THOROUGHLY TRACKED.

THE ADMINISTRATION STAFF KEEPS THE FAMILY UPDATED ON THE PROGRESS OF THE PATIENT, AND WHEN SOME MILESTONES ARE CROSSED. THE DOCTOR AND PSYCHIATRIST ALSO ROUTINELY UPDATE THE FAMILY ON THE PATIENTS WELL-BEING.

THE DEDICATED COUNSELLOR WORKS ALONGSIDE THE FAMILY MEMBERS TO CONDUCT FAMILY MEETINGS AND CONFRONTATIONS, BASED ON THE RECOVERY PROGRESS OF THE PATIENT.

THE FAMILY IS FREE TO CALL THE CENTRE TO SEEK UPDATES OR PROVIDE ANY ADDITIONAL CASE INFORMATION, BASED ON A CONVENIENT TIME SLOT FIXED WITH THE ADMINISTRATION OFFICE.

ANMOLJEEVANWELNESS@GMAIL.COM

WWW.ANMOLWELNESS.ORG

+91 915807 1666 / 915807 9666 &

+91 8080 8989 41/42

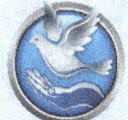 ANMOL JEEVAN FOUNDATION – PSYCHIATRIC HOSPITAL & NURSING HOME SPECIALIZED IN DE-ADDICTION THERAPY, MENTAL ILLNESS AND PSYCHIATRIC CARE – PERMANENT REGISTRATION NO. 5/2023

FEES, CHARGES, TERMS & CONDITIONS –

THE 45 DAY ACCELERATED RECOVERY PROGRAM IS AN ALL-INCLUSIVE PACKAGE, WITH SOME ITEMS THAT ARE SEPARATELY PAYABLE –

45 DAY PACKAGE ENROLMENT REQUIRES AN ADVANCE PAYMENT OF INR 60,000/-. THIS FEE IS PAYABLE FULLY IN ADVANCE. THESE FEES ARE NON-REFUNDABLE ON A PRORATED BASIS, AND THE ENTIRE PROGRAM MAY BE RE-ENROLLED BY PAYING THE SAME AMOUNT.

THIS FEE INCLUDES –

- THE DETOXIFICATION FEE + ONE ECG
- RESIDENT DOCTOR CHARGES
- PSYCHIATRIC DOCTOR CHARGES
- ONE ROUND OF BLOOD PANEL TESTING – (COMPLETE BLOOD COUNT, LIVER FUNCTION TEST, KIDNEY FUNCTION TEST, BLOOD-SUGAR TESTING & THYROID FUNCTION TEST)
- NARCO-URINE PLATE ANALYSIS
- ACCOMMODATION (AS DESCRIBED ABOVE)
- 3 SQUARE MEALS, AND EVENING SNACKS. SPECIAL MEALS ON WEEKENDS AND HOLIDAYS
- IN-ROOM SNACKS FOR ODD HOUR HUNGER PANGS
- LAUNDRY SERVICE
- ACCESS TO ALL AMENITIES SUCH AS THE SALON & SPA, GYMNASIUM, LIBRARY AND SPORTS / GAMES FACILITIES
- STATIONARY, STEP WORKING BOOK CHARGES, LAEFLETS, BOOKS AND INFORMATIONAL MATERIAL
- PSYCHOTHERAPY SESSIONS
- PSYCHOLOGICAL TESTING, REPORTING AND ANALYSIS
- COUNSELLOR & GUEST LECTURES
- INDIVIDUAL & GROUP COUNSELLING / THERAPY SESSIONS
- BASIC TOILETRIES (COMPRISING OF SHOWER GEL, SHAMPOO, TOOTHBRUSH / PASTE, DEODORANT)

ADDITIONAL CHARGES SHALL BE LEVIED FOR –

- ALL PRESCRIBED PHARMACEUTICALS, MEDICINES, CREAMS, LOTIONS ETC.
- PATIENT PICKUP MAY BE ARRANGED BY ANMOL JEEVAN, BUT SHALL BE CHARGED SEPARATELY
- ANY ADDITIONAL TESTS REQUIRED APART FROM THE ONES MENTIONED ABOVE
- X-RAYS, MRI, OR OTHER BLOOD, URINE AND STOOL TESTS
- ANY NON-PSYCHIATRIC CONSULTATION SUCH AS (BUT NOT LIMITED TO) ORTHOPAEDIC, OPHTHALMOLOGIST, DENTIST, UROLOGIST OR HEPATOLOGIST. ANMOL JEEVAN HAS STRATEGIC TIE-UPS FOR SUCH TESTS OR SPECIALIST CONSULTATIONS – THEY SHALL BE CHARGED ON ACTUALS
- ADDITIONAL CHARGES ON ACTUALS FOR SPECIFIC DEMANDS FOR TOILETRIES BEYOND THOSE MENTIONED ABOVE
- SPECIALITY FOOD TO BE ORDERED FROM OUTSIDE SHALL BE CHARGED ON ACTUALS
- AMBULANCE FEES FOR TRANSPORTATION SHALL BE SEPARATELY CHARGED

© 2023 - A WELLBEING GUIDE FOR THE FAMILIES & FRIENDS OF ALCOHOL, DRUG, SEX ADDICTS, AND COMPULSIVE GAMBLERS BY THE ANMOL JEEVAN FOUNDATION™
ANMOLJEEVANWELNESS@GMAIL.COM WWW.ANMOLWELNESS.ORG
+91 915807 1666 / 915807 9666 & +91 8080 8989 41/42

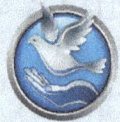 ANMOL JEEVAN FOUNDATION – PSYCHIATRIC HOSPITAL & NURSING HOME SPECIALIZED IN DE-ADDICTION THERAPY, MENTAL ILLNESS AND PSYCHIATRIC CARE – PERMANENT REGISTRATION NO. 5/2023

THANK YOU

WE WISH YOU THE BEST IN ALL YOUR ENDEAVOURS

MAY YOU ALWAYS PROSPER – THE RIGHT WAY!

AT ANMOL JEEVAN WELLNESS – <u>WE ARE FRIENDS TO THE FALLEN</u> AND GUIDES TO THOSE ON THE PATH OF RECOVERY. IT IS OUR STRONGEST BELIEF THAT EVERYONE CAN RESTORE THEIR LIVES TO THE FULLEST, NO MATTER WHAT THEIR PAST HAS BEEN. <u>WE HAVE THE FAITH THAT NO LOSS CAN BE BIG ENOUGH TO LOOSE ALL HOPE</u>; AND ALL BAD TIMES SHALL PASS – BY GOD'S GRACE.

© 2023 - A WELLBEING GUIDE FOR THE FAMILIES & FRIENDS OF ALCOHOL, DRUG, SEX ADDICTS, AND COMPULSIVE GAMBLERS BY THE ANMOL JEEVAN FOUNDATION™
ANMOLJEEVANWELNESS@GMAIL.COM WWW.ANMOLWELNESS.ORG
+91 915807 1666 / 915807 9666 & +91 8080 8989 41/42

www.ingramcontent.com/pod-product-compliance
Lightning Source LLC
Chambersburg PA
CBHW082208220526
45470CB00010B/3086